ADVANCES IN HEALTH AND DISEASE

VOLUME 4

ADVANCES IN HEALTH AND DISEASE

Additional books in this series can be found on Nova's website under the Series tab.

Additional e-books in this series can be found on Nova's website under the eBooks tab.

ADVANCES IN HEALTH AND DISEASE

ADVANCES IN HEALTH AND DISEASE

VOLUME 4

LOWELL T. DUNCAN
EDITOR

nova biomedical
New York

Library of Congress Cataloging-in-Publication Data

ISBN: 978-1-53613-345-5

Published by Nova Science Publishers, Inc. † New York

Contents

PREFACE

In *Advances in Health and Disease. Volume 4*, the authors open by reflecting on the potential advantages and challenges of the focus group technique in health services research, based on a study conducted to better understand the perceptions and experiences related to access and utilization of healthcare services for immigrants in Portugal. Later, the authors examine Parvovirus B19 (PVB19), a widespread infection that affects 1-5% of pregnant women. The authors maintain that as PVB19 infection can cause severe morbidity and mortality, it should be part of the routine work up of complicated pregnancies, especially when fetal hydrops is suspected. This book also summarizes the evidence on propensity for TDM in anti-TNF therapy to guide interventions at therapeutic failure, while present data do not support the routine use of proactive TDM in everyday clinical practice. The authors maintain that the use of statins is necessary for the prevention and treatment of atherosclerosis, and the criteria for assessing their hypolipidemic effect are clearly defined. Depending on the severity of experimental hyperlipoproteinemia, oral administration of atorvastatin may have a different effect on the overall activity of MMPs in the serum of mice. The following chapter discusses how employing focus groups provided the opportunity to 1) check cultural assumptions, 2) assess and prioritize areas of greatest perceived need, 3) tailor campaigns and outreach to the key values and beliefs of the population of focus, and 4) understand and capitalize on social media and other communication favored by Hispanic young adults in a minority serving institution in order to reduce HIV related health disparities. Next, Congenital Hypothyroidism is examined as the most common endocrine disorder in childhood. In the last years the decrease of the TSH recall threshold has led to an increased of mild forms with *in situ* glands at the first diagnosis. As such, the re-evaluation of the diagnosis has become an important procedure to distinguish transient forms from permanent ones. Three types of Burkitt's Lymphoma are also examined, including Endemic (African), Sporadic (non-African) and HIV-associated per WHO classification. Compared to the endemic type which is commonly associated with EBV infection, the incidence of EBV is lower in the other two types (20% in sporadic and 30- 40% in HIV patients). After which, end stage renal disease is examined in the same manner, reviewing the diagnosis, management and consequences. In a separate study, an integrated mixed method approach was used in 5 coastal communities in Tongatapu, Tonga, where some community members had their health and well-being affected by climate change and some did not. Results indicated that physical, mental and spiritual aspects of well-being were affected by climate change and that people were eager to see the implementation of strategies to improve their health and restore their mental well-being. The concluding study aimed to verify the influence of different motivational interventions for oral hygiene autonomy promotion on the biofilm control in individuals with special needs. The data suggest that motivational activities can be developed to promote autonomy in other aspects of general health, resulting in the improvement of the quality of life of individuals with special needs.

Chapter 1 - Focus groups have been widely used in health research to explore the perspectives and experiences of individuals regarding health, illness and the health system, and to understand its sociocultural and contextual factors. Migrant health is increasingly a research topic of interest nationwide. Immigrants are recognized as a group that tends to underuse healthcare services, which has a negative impact on their health and their integration into the host society. Research on migrants' access to and utilization of healthcare services has been based mainly on quantitative data. However, qualitative research through focus groups may contribute to gain a deeper understanding of the challenges that migrant populations face in seeking healthcare. In this chapter the authors reflect on the potential, advantages and challenges of the focus group technique in health services research, based on a study which was conducted to understand better the perceptions and experiences related to access and utilization of healthcare services of immigrants in Portugal; the study examines the data from the perspectives of the immigrants as well as health workers. Six focus groups were conducted with 20 immigrant community leaders and 32 health workers. The authors first contextualize the study and then focus on the use of the focus group technique, because of its potential for providing rich and valuable information within a diverse cultural setting. Furthermore, focus groups contribute with dynamic ideas and discussion, which do not arise from individual interviews. Then the authors describe the process of cattying out the focus groups. The focus group dynamic stimulated lively discussions around access and utilization of healthcare services among immigrant populations. Participants shared their experiences and views, and expressed their disagreements with factors influencing migrants' access and utilization of health services. Finally, the authors debate the strengths as well as the challenges of using this technique. The focus group dynamics helped eliminate defensive attitudes regarding, for example, immigrants' legal status. However, the sensitive nature of this topic and the potential effect of group interaction may have inhibited the disclosure of experiences and perceptions of some participants, especially among the health workers, regarding the denial of care to undocumented immigrants. Overall, during the focus group sessions, participants were not merely "study subjects" but could actively participate in the process of reflecting on proposals for overcoming the identified barriers and improving access and utilization of health services among immigrants. The use of focus group technique was valuable in that it produced better knowledge on the real health needs of immigrants and health workers in their daily lives, increased awareness on the topic and helped identify opportunities for effective action.

Chapter 2 - Parvovirus B19 (PVB19) is a widespread infection that may affects 1-5% of pregnant women; in epidemics, the rate of infection is even higher. In spite of 30%- 50% vertical transmission to the fetus, pregnancy outcome is generally unaffected. Diagnosis of infection is by maternal serology and/or PCR, but fetal infection is diagnosed by PCR from amniotic fluid or, if fetal cordocentesis is carried out, from fetal blood. Reports on major congenital anomalies among offspring of mothers infected by Parvovirus B19 affecting different organs are scanty, as the virus does not seem to be a significant human teratogen. However, especially if infection occurs in the first half of pregnancy, it may cause significant fetal damage and rarely also brain anomalies and neurodevelopmental problems. PVB19 is an important cause of fetal loss throughout gestation, especially in the second half of pregnancy; at that time spontaneous fetal loss from other causes is relatively rare. The virus infects fetal erythroid progenitor cells causing apoptosis and, as a result of shortened half-life of erythrocytes moderate to severe fetal anemia. Severe thrombocytopenia is also common. According to its severity, the anemia may lead to high output cardiac failure and therefore non immune hydrops fetalis (NIHF). PVB19 may also directly infect myocardial cells and produce myocarditis that aggravates the cardiac failure. Intrauterine fetal transfusion, which is commonly carried out for the treatment of severe fetal anemia, significantly reduces fetal morbidity. There are little data regarding the long-term neurodevelopmental outcome in infected children. Although data are inadequate, 10-15% of the children infected with PVB19 having hydrops fetalis will suffer from neurodevelopmental impairment. However, there seem to be no data on infected fetuses without hydrops. It is also unknown whether neurodevelopmental sequelae result from the anemia or from the complications of the intrauterine transfusion, since children who had fetal hydrops and intrauterine transfusion due to other etiologies were also found to have a high rate of neurodevelopmental problems. Since PVB19 infection can cause severe morbidity and mortality, it should be part of the routine work up of complicated pregnancies, especially when fetal hydrops is suspected. Risk assessment for maternal infection during pregnancy is particularly important during epidemics when sero-conversion rates are high. Until today, there is no effective immunization against parvovirus.

Chapter 3 - Over the past 15 years, tumor necrosis factor (TNF) antagonists have revolutionized therapy for inflammatory bowel disease

(IBD). Yet, a significant proportion of patients does not respond or lose effect to anti-TNF therapy over time. A 'tailored' treatment approach for anti-TNF treatment optimization has been suggested. Patient characterization is important prior and during therapy, multiple factors should be evaluated including clinical and disease characteristics, genetic factors and therapeutic drug monitoring (TDM) measuring anti-TNF drug levels and anti-drug antibodies (ADA). TDM can aid therapeutic decisions during primary and secondary treatment failure to anti-TNF treatment or proactive optimization of long-term disease management. TDM is routinely applied in the evaluation of secondary loss of response. The TDM-based strategy has several advantages over an empiric approach as it avoids unnecessary dose intensification, allows targeted switching between anti-TNF agents or out of class, and optimizes health care resources. Proactive TDM-based strategy to prevent anti-TNF treatment failure has also been suggested/investigated. However, routine monitoring of trough anti-TNF drug concentrations and targeted dose optimization had no additional benefit with regards to 1-year clinical outcome over strict clinical/biochemical based patient monitoring as observed in the TAXIT and TAILORIX trials. Of note, the TDM-based strategy of the TAXIT trial was associated with significantly fewer disease flares. Emerging data are published from real life cohorts, including, e.g., Belgium, The Netherlands, U.S., Denmark, France and Hungary supporting the case for TDM assessment at loss of response leading to earlier optimization of medical therapy and cost reduction, while further evidence is needed on the additional value of proactive TDM. This book chapter summarizes the evidence on the use of TDM in anti-TNF therapy to guide interventions at therapeutic failure, while present data do not support the routine use of proactive TDM in everyday clinical practice.

Chapter 4 - The use of statins is necessary for the prevention and treatment of atherosclerosis, and the criteria for assessing their hypolipidemic effect are clearly defined. Atorvastatin is one of the most commonly prescribed statins in cardiology and other branches of clinical medicine. The pleiotropic effects of statins have not been thoroughly studied until now. In clinical practice, results of a high-sensitivity C-reactive protein (hs-CRP) assay, which reflect the anti-inflammatory effect of various drugs, are commonly analyzed. It appears to be relevant at present to evaluate the effects of statins on changes in new biochemical markers of a nonlipid nature that reflect the progression of atherosclerosis and the involvement of activated macrophages in the pathogenesis. Atorvastatin treatment of patients with ischemic heart disease and atherosclerosis decreases serum hs-CRP results and serum interleukin 6 and TNF-α concentrations. It was noted that the use of statins decreases both the activity and expression of matrix metalloproteases (MMPs) in atherosclerotic plaques. Although high levels of low-density lipoprotein (LDL)-cholesterol, low levels of HDL-cholesterol, and increased activity of MMPs are common risk factors for ischemic heart disease, it remains unclear how the activities of other possible biomarkers of nonlipid nature (like chitotriosidase, MMPs, and the concentration of cystatin C) change at different stages of the disease and during treatment with atorvastatin. Therefore, it would be worthwhile to evaluate the changes in the activity of chitotriosidase and MMPs and a cystatin C concentration in relation to both lipid indices and changes in hs-CRP results in the serum of patients with atherosclerosis and those who are being treated with statins, especially after myocardial revascularization by a coronary bypass. It has been shown experimentally that, depending on the severity of experimental hyperlipoproteinemia, oral administration of atorvastatin has a different effect on the overall activity of MMPs in the serum of mice. An increase in the activity of chitotriosidase in the serum of atorvastatin-treated mice is known to be independent of the severity of experimental hyperlipoproteinemia, whereas changes in the activity of MMPs during atorvastatin treatment positively correlate with the severity of experimentally induced hyperlipoproteinemia.

Chapter 5 - Community-based research (CBR) methods are essential for addressing the social, structural, and environmental factors that contribute to health disparities among underrepresented yet disproportionately affected minority groups. CBR enriches project implementation and the research process by involving community members in all project phases, leading to insights and health enhancements, and program sustainability not otherwise obtainable. Research aimed at alleviating persistent health disparities, particularly targeting behavioral health and preventable diseases, requires deliberate and direct involvement of the population of interest in order to be most effective and promote sustained change. In CBR, key stakeholders are actively involved and engaged in the research process from the start. These stakeholders have a direct impact on the decisions made in the design, implementation, and evaluation of projects. Conducting focus groups can be an effective way to involve the population of interest in the research process. Focus groups give community members the opportunity to recount experiences, share insights, and engage in dialogue with other community members and the researchers with whom they are partnering. Focus groups can be particularly helpful when dealing with racial, ethnic or sexual minority groups, whose experiences often do not mirror the experiences of those from the dominant culture. Furthermore, focus groups can inform researchers about how specific minority subgroups of individuals receive and exchange health information that they find credible and impactful. Such knowledge is critical for the successful dissemination of health information using social media and networking technologies, given the fast pace of change and the immense popularity of these communication tools among young adults. Focus groups can help ensure that the needs of underrepresented and rapidly changing populations are understood, that projects are culturally and linguistically appropriate and relevant, and that trust and communication between researchers and community members is established and maintained. This chapter describes focus groups conducted as part of a federally-funded University CBR partnership program for preventing HIV and substance abuse among Hispanic emerging adults in Miami-Dade County. Miami-Dade County has the highest rates of HIV infection in the U. S. Using a real-world example, this chapter will discuss how employing focus groups provided the opportunity to 1) check cultural assumptions, 2) assess and prioritize areas of greatest perceived need, 3) tailor campaigns and outreach to the key values and beliefs of population of focus, and 4) understand and capitalize on social media and other communication favored by the population of focus to reduce health disparities. This chapter also offer suggestions as to how focus groups can be used as an instrumental technique to contributing to the success of CBR partnerships aimed at promoting health equity and alleviating health disparities, specifically related to HIV, among minority communities.

Chapter 6 - Background: Congenital Hypothyroidism (CH) is the most common endocrine disorder in childhood. Levothyroxine treatment within the first 2-3 weeks of life prevent neurological damage. Newborn screening (NS) by TSH dosage on dried blood spot allowed to early identification of risk for CH. In the last years the reduction of TSH recall threshold has led to an increased detection of mild forms with in situ gland at the first diagnosis. Therefore, the re-evaluation of diagnosis has become an important procedure to distingue transient forms from permanent ones. *Aetiology:* Transient CH may be caused by maternal factors (deficiency/excess of iodine, TSH receptor blockers, drugs) or neonatal factors (preterm and NICU infants; heterozygous mutations of the DUOX2 and DUOXA2 genes). *Epidemiology:* Before NS, the incidence of CH was 1:7000-10000 live births. After the introduction of NS it increased to 1:3000-4000. Currently, it is 1:1600-2800. This increase is correlated with the lowering TSH recall threshold, the increase in multiple pregnancies and preterm infants, and demographic changes. *Re-evaluation of CH:* it is performed after third year of life. According to the European guidelines, two different strategies can be adopted: the discontinuation of therapy over a period of 4-6 weeks or by decreasing the dose of Levothyroxine by 30% for 2–3 weeks followed by the dosing of serum levels of TSH and fT4. CH is permanent if an increase in TSH ≥ 10 mU/L is demonstrated. The etiology of CH can be identified using thyroid ultrasound (US), Iodine-123 scintigraphy, and in selected cases the perchlorate test. If the US shows a normal thyroid volume and scintigraphy shows low/absent tracer uptake, TSH resistance is presumable. If the US shows a normal or increased volume of thyroid, with a greedy absorption of the tracer to scintigraphy, dyshormonogenesis by the perchlorate test could be investigated. A radiolabel wash out of 10% of baseline uptake 2 hours after administration of perchlorate is indicative of a defect in organification (partial with a wash out between 10-90%; total with a wash out >90%). The US findings of a normal or increased thyroid volume associated with high TSH and very low/unmeasurable thyroglobulin levels point to a deficiency of thyroglobulin synthesis. In the authors' regional program of NS in the last ten years 491/454024 children were recalled for TSH and the diagnosis of CH was confirmed in 82.5%. The incidence of CH was 1:1121 births. 280 patients showed CH with *in situ* gland. After re-evaluation of diagnosis a permanent form of CH was detected in 55% of the cases (29% with hyperthyrotropinemia). A partial form of organification defect was detected in 34.5% of subjects submitted to perchlorate test and a TSH resistance due to a heterozygous mutation of the TSH-receptor gene was detected in 28.6%. Birth at term, the thyroid hypoplasia and a higher therapeutic dose of Levothyroxine (>2 mcg/Kg) at the re-evaluation were predictive factors of a permanent form. The frequent persistence of thyroid dysfunction in patients with borderline TSH values at the NS underlines the importance of reducing the recall threshold.

Chapter 7 - *Etiology:* There are three types of Burkitt's Lymphoma: Endemic (African), Sporadic (non-African) and HIV-associated per WHO classification. Compared to the endemic type which is commonly associated with EBV infection, the incidence of EBV is lower in the other two types (20% in sporadic and 30- 40% in HIV patients). Burkitt's Lymphoma is distinguished from diffuse large-B-cell lymphoma by the high level of expression of c-myc, the expression of germinal-center B-cell genes, and the low level of MHC class I genes and nuclear factor-kappa target genes. Immunodeficiency-associated Burkitt's lymphoma occurs mainly in patients infected with HIV but also occurs in allograft recipients and individuals with congenital immunodeficiency. Burkitt's lymphoma accounts for 30%–40% of non-Hodgkin's lymphoma in HIV+ patients. Burkitt's lymphoma is estimated to be 1,000 times more common in HIV+ individuals. HIV+ patients with Burkitt's lymphoma are younger, less often carry a prior diagnosis of AIDS, and have higher mean CD4 counts. HIV-associated Burkitt's lymphoma shares some pathogenetic features with endemic Burkitt's lymphoma. Patients with Burkitt's lymphoma have a median age of 54.5 years with a CR rate of 72% and a lymphoma free long-time survival of 55%. The International Prognostic Index IPI is the most valuable prognostic factor for survival. Favorable disease by Murphy's system is stage I or stage IIR and normal LDH. *Symptoms:* Endemic Burkitt's lymphoma most commonly involves the maxilla and/or mandible; however, abdominal organs may also be involved. A tumor can double in size in 18 hours. Presentation is commonly with swelling of the affected jaw bones and rapidly enlarging, non-tender lymph nodes in the neck or jaw. Sporadic Burkitt's lymphoma usually involves the abdominal organs, most frequently the distal ileum, caecum or mesentery. Other abdominal and pelvic organs, glandular tissue (such as the thyroid and tonsils) and the facial bones may also be involved. Presentation is commonly with abdominal mass/swelling and ascites, intestinal obstruction. B symptoms may be present with both forms of Burkitt's lymphoma and include fever, weight loss, night sweats. HIV-related Burkitt's lymphoma tends to present in a similar way to the sporadic disease. *Treatment Options:* Treatment of Burkitt's lymphoma in younger and fit patients is R-HyperCVAD, R-CODOX/MVAC. For low-risk disease with single site of disease <10 cm and a normal LDH, 3 cycles of R-CODOX-M are considered. For older patients more than 60 years of age R-EPOCH is preferred but R-HyperCVAD could be considered for select older fit patients. Salvage chemotherapy options for relapsed Burkitt's lymphoma are aggressive CCE or other ALL induction regimens. Allogeneic transplants may be considered for fit patients who obtain second CR. The patient should receive CNS prophylaxis with each cycle of chemotherapy. For HIV-related Burkitt's lymphoma, a dose-Adjusted R-EPOCH is again considered a preferred treatment. For young, fit patients with well-controlled HIV and good $CD4^+$ counts R-HyperCVAD and R-CODOX-M/IVAC could be considered as alternative treatment options. The overall survival is superior among those who receive intensive chemotherapy regimens instead of lower-dose regimens.

Chapter 8 - Extremes of blood pressure are not uncommon in end stage renal disease (ESRD) patients that are associated with increased morbidities and mortalities. The authors will review the diagnosis, management and consequences of these in this chapter. Interdialytic ambulatory blood pressure (ABP) or home BP, especially after the mid-week dialysis including the weekend, is the gold standard in diagnosis of hypertension in dialysis patients. Interdialytic ASBP of >130 mmHg or home SBP of >140 mmHg is associated with poor outcomes including mortality. Lowering of elevated

BP in dialysis patients has shown to be beneficial. Treatment includes non-pharmacological measures, such as enhanced sodium removal with dialysis, dietary sodium restriction, probing of dry weight, prolonged dialysis duration and intensive dialysis treatment, and pharmacological measures. Selection of antihypertensive medications should take into consideration of underlying co-morbidities of the individuals, side effect profiles, and intra- and inter-dialytic pharmacokinetics of the medications. Beta-blocker is the preferred drug class among ESRD population due to its cardiovascular benefits. Low dialyzable beta-blockers are shown to have better mortality benefits than highly dialyzable ones. Calcium channel blockers, Angiotensin converting enzyme inhibitors and Angiotensin receptor blockers are also effective antihypertensive agents. Centrally acting alpha-agonist, direct vasodilators, and alpha-adrenergic blockers are adjunctive agents that are generally recommended for multidrug-resistant hypertension due to unfavorable side-effects and adherence concerns. Usage of mineralocorticoid receptor antagonists as antihypertensive agent is limited due to risk of hyperkalemia, but it is shown to minimize cardiovascular events in some studies. More data will be available after the completion of ALCHEMIST and SPin-D trials. At the other end of the blood pressure spectrum, hypotension during or immediately following dialysis is an equally common phenomenon. Intradialytic hypotension (IDH) is defined by KDOQI guidelines as "a decrease systolic blood pressure by ≥20 mm Hg or a decrease in MAP by 10 mm Hg associated with symptoms." IDH carries a host of complications, including dysrhythmias, cardiac and cerebral ischemia, and fluid overload related to difficult ultrafiltration. It has been well known that there is "U"-shaped curve relationship between post-dialysis SBP and CV mortality in ESRD patients. The risk factors for IDH include extremes of age, diabetics, cardiac dysfunction, coronary heart disease, and large interdialytic weight gains. Although IDH may occur due to serious underlying medical conditions, often no such causes are identified. The acute management of IDH consists of immediate reduction or discontinuation of ultrafiltration, administration of fluid bolus and oxygen, Trendelenburg position to increase cerebral perfusion. Long term conservative management of IDH encompasses reassessment of estimated dry weight, withholding antihypertensives before dialysis treatment, avoiding food intake just before and during dialysis, avoidance of large intradialytic weight gain, cool-temperature dialysate, use of midodrine, longer dialysis duration to allow for gentler ultrafiltration. In addition to these conservative measures, patients with persistent IDH will need a cardiac evaluation, including an echocardiogram.

Chapter 9 - Understanding the perceptions of climate change impacts on people's health and well-being in coastal communities is essential to develop adaptation strategies that will improve the health and well-being of community members in coastal areas. Here, an integrated mixed method approach: concurrent convergence parallel triangulation design – was used in 5 coastal communities in Tongatapu, Tonga. Community members were interviewed. Some of them had their health and well-being affected by climate change and some were not affected. Their responses were analyzed using a non-parametric test – chi-square analysis. Themes regarding the impact of climate change on health and well-being were then used to generate a further hypothesis. The results show that those whose health and well-being was affected differed significantly from those who were unaffected. They also indicated that all aspects of well-being: physical, mental and spiritual were affected by climate change and that people were eager to see the implementation of climate change adaptation strategies to improve their health and restore their mental well-being. It is thus essential to include these issues in adaptation strategies to ensure that local people are supporting and taking ownership of their resilience building.

Chapter 10 - This study aimed to verify the influence of different motivational interventions for oral hygiene autonomy promotion on the biofilm control in individuals with special needs. The study sample consisted of 21 adult individuals with mean age of 30 years, with several types of disabilities (cerebral palsy, Down syndrome, intellectual retarded, and autism), employees of the sector of artisan products of the Universidade Metodista de São Paulo. The biofilm was evaluated through the Simplified Oral Hygiene Index (OHI-S) proposed by Greene and Vermillion (1964). None of the participants (0%) exhibited excellent or bad initial values of oral hygiene; 80.95% exhibited good and 19.05% regular initial values. Then, four different types of motivational activities on oral health were carried out for 4 months. The following percentages of the values of oral hygiene after the first motivational activity (motivational theater) were observed: excellent and bad 0%, good 66.7%, and regular 33.33%. After the second motivational activity (group dynamics with sequence of tooth brushing play, none of the participants presented excellent OHI-S, while 23.8% scored regular, 71.4% good and 4.8% bad. In the motivational activity of supervised tooth brushing, the authors verified an increasing of good OHI-S (90.4%) and a decreasing for regular OHI-S (9.6%). The last motivational intervention was a talk with parents and/or guardians and the OHI-S analysis showed that 4.8% reached an excellent score, 90.4% a good score, 4.8% a regular score and 0% a bad score. The Friedman test ($p<0.005$) revealed statistically significant differences in the comparison between the 1st and 5th; 2nd and 4th; 2nd and 5th; 3rd and 4th; and 3rd and 5th OHI-S assessments. It was concluded that the oral hygiene promotion autonomy in individuals with special needs can be effective, especially when a continuous and individualized following-up is possible in addition to the motivation of parents and/or guardians. Thus, OHI-S decreased, ensuring an improvement in oral health. These data suggest that motivational activities can be developed to promote autonomy in other aspects of general health, resulting in the improvement of the quality of life of individuals with special needs.

In: Advances in Health and Disease. Volume 4 ISBN: 978-1-53613-345-5
Editor: Lowell T. Duncan

Chapter 1

THE POTENTIAL OF FOCUS GROUPS IN HEALTH RESEARCH: A STUDY ON IMMIGRANTS' ACCESS TO AND UTILIZATION OF HEALTH SERVICES

Sónia Dias*[*], *PhD and Ana Gama
Global Health and Tropical Medicine, GHTM, Instituto de Higiene e Medicina Tropical, IHMT, Universidade Nova de Lisboa, UNL, Lisboa, Portugal

ABSTRACT

Focus groups have been widely used in health research to explore the perspectives and experiences of individuals regarding health, illness and the health system, and to understand its sociocultural and contextual factors. Migrant health is increasingly a research topic of interest nationwide. Immigrants are recognized as a group that tends to underuse healthcare services, which has a negative impact on their health and their integration into the host society. Research on migrants' access to and

[*] Corresponding Author Email: smfdias@yahoo.com.

utilization of healthcare services has been based mainly on quantitative data. However, qualitative research through focus groups may contribute to gain a deeper understanding of the challenges that migrant populations face in seeking healthcare. In this chapter we reflect on the potential, advantages and challenges of the focus group technique in health services research, based on a study which was conducted to understand better the perceptions and experiences related to access and utilization of healthcare services of immigrants in Portugal; the study examines the data from the perspectives of the immigrants as well as health workers. Six focus groups were conducted with 20 immigrant community leaders and 32 health workers. We first contextualize the study and then focus on the use of the focus group technique, because of its potential for providing rich and valuable information within a diverse cultural setting. Furthermore, focus groups contribute with dynamic ideas and discussion, which do not arise from individual interviews. Then we describe the process of cattying out the focus groups. The focus group dynamic stimulated lively discussions around access and utilization of healthcare services among immigrant populations. Participants shared their experiences and views, and expressed their disagreements with factors influencing migrants' access and utilization of health services. Finally, we debate the strengths as well as the challenges of using this technique. The focus group dynamics helped eliminate defensive attitudes regarding, for example, immigrants' legal status. However, the sensitive nature of this topic and the potential effect of group interaction may have inhibited the disclosure of experiences and perceptions of some participants, especially among the health workers, regarding the denial of care to undocumented immigrants. Overall, during the focus group sessions, participants were not merely "study subjects" but could actively participate in the process of reflecting on proposals for overcoming the identified barriers and improving access and utilization of health services among immigrants. The use of focus group technique was valuable in that it produced better knowledge on the real health needs of immigrants and health workers in their daily lives, increased awareness on the topic and helped identify opportunities for effective action.

Keywords: focus groups, health research, immigrants, health workers

INTRODUCTION

The focus group is a research technique for the collection of qualitative information from groups of participants through discussion sessions regarding specific topics proposed by a moderator (Fern, 2001; Krueger &

Casey, 2000; Morgan, 2001). The main goal of a focus group is to explore personal experiences, beliefs, attitudes and values underlying a theme through the opinions expressed by participants individually and collectively (Fern, 2001; Krueger & Casey, 2000). This technique is considered extremely useful to understand concepts, vocabulary patterns and thoughts of a certain population inserted in a social context (Barbour & Kitzinger, 1999; Goldman & Schmalz, 2001; Hollander, 2004; Rich & Ginsburg, 1999). It allows access to participants' cognitive, emotional and social models and also the processes of production of associated meanings, perceptions, attitudes and actions (Hyde et al., 2005; Morgan, 2001). As documented in the literature, this technique gathers information not only about individuals' behaviour, but also about the social, cultural and political context influencing it (Dias, Matos & Gonçalves, 2001; Dias, Matos & Gonçalves, 2002; Frith, 2000; Goldman & Schmalz, 2001; Hollander, 2004; Krueger & Casey, 2000).

The focus group has become a popular technique for data collection which is widely used in social sciences and specifically in health care research (Halcomb et al., 2007; Kitzinger, 2000; Lobdell et al., 2005; Peterson-Sweeney, 2005). The use of this technique is intended to promote better understanding of the multiple variables that contribute to the complex, and often contradictory, belief systems, attitudes, lifestyles, and risk factors related to health, as they develop within a social, economic and cultural context characterized by the specific reality of the individuals. In the context of health promotion and disease prevention, this technique can be an effective means to determine significant beliefs and opinions impacting the decision to adopt certain health behaviours. It is especially efficient in the identification of barriers preventing or discouraging individuals from embracing healthy behaviours (Green & Thorogood, 2004; Linhorst, 2002).

Indeed, a set of multiple, complex, and interrelated social determinants influence health behaviours and health status, shaping populations' health vulnerability (Davies, Basten & Frattini, 2009). In the context of increasing migration in Europe, the health status of immigrant populations has been of great concern for several decades (World Health Organization, 2010). Health is recognised as a critical factor for migrants' well-being as well as better integration into the host country (Ingleby et al. 2005; Peiro & Benedict 2009).

The migration of people from many different cultural and ethnic backgrounds into Europe has become a common phenomenon; a total of 4.7 million people migrated to one of the European Union Member States during 2015 (Eurostat, 2017). In Portugal, 397,731 foreign citizens were residing legally in 2016, mainly from Brazil, Portuguese-speaking African countries and Eastern European countries (Serviço de Estrangeiros e Fronteiras, 2017).

When leaving their country of origin, migrants are usually healthier than the native-born citizens of the host country - the alleged “healthy migrant” effect (Blair & Schneeberg, 2014; Kuerban, 2016). However, immigrants in various social, cultural and political contexts report poorer self-perceived health when compared with the general population (Giannoni, Franzini & Masiero, 2016; Nielsen & Krasnik, 2010; Rechel et al., 2013). In fact, migrants may face increased risk factors such as poor living and working conditions, separation from social and family networks, and social exclusion, making them more vulnerable to injuries, non-communicable and communicable diseases, mental health problems and psychological stress (Rechel et al., 2013).

Access and utilization of health services by immigrant populations are important for the reduction of morbidity, positive health outcomes and integration into the host country (Kristiansen, Mygind & Krasnik, 2007; Nordhaus, 2002; Politzer et al., 2001; Solar & Irwin, 2007; World Health Organization, 2007). Health is recognized as a universal human right (World Health Organization, 1948) and the pursuit of equity in access to health services has been a main goal of healthcare systems. However, inequities persist in health services access and their use by immigrant populations (Buja et al., 2013; Dias, Severo & Barros, 2008; Goddard & Smith 2001; Hargreaves et al., 2006; Muennig & Fahs 2002; Quan et al. 2006). Indeed, several studies indicate that migrant populations are not always covered by health care systems in the host countries in terms of disease prevention, treatment and health promotion. When compared to native populations, immigrant populations tend to present lower rates of health services utilization (Dias, Severo & Barros, 2008; Graetz et al., 2017; Machado et al., 2006; Muennig & Fahs, 2002; Norredam, Nielsen & Krasnik, 2010; Quan et al., 2006).

Several factors may impact migrant's access and use of healthcare services. Migrants' socioeconomic characteristics, such as educational level, employment status, economic status and financial resources may hinder their access to care (Dias, Severo & Barros, 2008; Scheppers et al., 2006). Undocumented status can also translate into more difficulties in getting medical assistance (Dias et al., 2011a; Graetz et al., 2017; Rechel et al., 2013). Other individual factors are based on cultural background and include beliefs and attitudes toward health/illness and expectations on healthcare (Scheppers et al., 2006). Other factors include gaps in health literacy, short length of residence in the host country and the associated lack of knowledge of how health services function (Rechel et al., 2013; Scheppers et al., 2006). On the other hand, healthcare professionals' attitudes toward migrants, insufficient cultural skills and language barriers may discourage migrants from seeking medical assistance (Dias et al., 2011b; Scheppers et al., 2006). Finally, health service schedules, infrastructure, bureaucratic procedures and costs also may limit migrants' access to healthcare (Giannoni, Franzini & Masiero, 2016; Rechel et al., 2013; Scheppers et al., 2006).

In Portugal, the Constitution establishes that every person has the right to healthcare services, regardless of nationality, legal status, socioeconomic status or any other criterion. Migrants have the same right to access the health system as Portuguese citizens (Simões et al., 2017); undocumented migrants must pay the full price of services, but fee exemptions are granted similarly to national citizens in cases of public health threats. Despite legislative support, a study with African, Brazilian and Eastern European migrants reported that only 77% used the National Health Service (Dias et al., 2011a).

A more comprehensive approach is needed to understand the barriers preventing migrants from accessing health services. In this context, this study explores the perspectives and experiences of both immigrants and health workers related to migrants' access to and use of health services, through a qualitative approach using the focus groups technique. The main purpose was to identify migrants' needs and to develop and implement strategies and policies oriented toward a more adequate provision of healthcare to migrants. In addition, the study aims to promote the access and utilization of health services, leading to effective health gain in these communities.

The decision to use focus groups in this study was based on the fact that migrants' access and utilization of health services are influenced by a complex combination of individual subjective features, socioeconomic factors and cultural structures, and the associated impacts that arise in complex social interactions (Hollander, 2004; Parker, Easton & Klein, 2000; Rechel et al., 2013; Scheppers et al., 2006). This technique was selected to provide a context in which to explore and clarify the way personal views are related to group perspectives. Furthermore, we explore how a collective perspective is interactive rather than fixed. Focus groups have been used extensively in research with migrants and culturally diverse groups (Dias et al., 2002; Halcomb et al., 2007), as well as with health professionals (Lester, Tritter & Sorohan, 2005).

METHODS

Study Design

A qualitative study using focus groups was conducted with migrants residing in Portugal and health workers.

Participants

There are no strict criteria for the definition of the number of participants in a focus group. Given that statistical representativeness is not the goal of this technique (Barbour & Kitzinger, 1999), a focus group usually involves a small number of people (between 6 and 12), depending on the purpose for which the group is constituted (Morgan, 2001). An optimal solution must ensure enough people so that discussion and differences of opinion occur. Just as the majority of the studies that use this method, the interest of this study was to explore the participants' perspectives, experiences and attitudes, rather than to seek generalizations. Several authors propose the creation of small groups when the topic of concern is of interest for participants and they are closely involved in the discussion, as was the case of this study (Kitzinger, 2000; Krueger & Casey, 2000). That way, every person has the opportunity to participate in the discussion, making it more rich and complete. Similarly, the number of groups for a certain study does not have to be exhaustive; yet every attempt is made to reach data saturation; saturation is achieved when no further ideas emerge from the data (Bowen, 2008; Houghton et al., 2013; O'Reilly & Parker, 2012). Also, the number of focus groups is highly dependent on logistic conditions (time, technical and human resources) for the data collection and analysis.

Generally, participants with shared characteristics are selected based on criteria relevant to the topic under study (Krueger & Casey, 2000). Sociodemographic homogeneity of the participants can facilitate communication within the group, but it does not mean homogeneity in attitudes, beliefs and behaviours. Indeed, the organization of the groups must be meticulous, in order to facilitate communication among the group, keeping the heterogeneity of attitudes, beliefs and behaviours (Farquhar & Das, 1999; Hyde et al., 2005; Kitzinger, 2000). On the subject of health, for example, the constitution of homogeneous groups with regard to sociodemographic characteristics, such as cultural background and socioeconomic level is generally recommended (Farquhar & Das, 1999; Kitzinger, 2000).

For this study, 20 migrants and 32 health workers were enrolled. Data were collected separately from migrants and health workers as a way to better understand the dual perspectives of those providing and receiving healthcare. For the focus groups with migrants, key informants in the communities were contacted and invited to participate in the study. This activity was developed in collaboration with NGOs and migrant associations. The inclusion criterion was to be a "migrant", defined as a foreign-born person that migrated to settle in Portugal (International Organization for Migration, 2004). Participants were also included according to their readiness and explicit interest in participating. Migrants originating from Portuguese-speaking African countries, Brazil and Eastern European countries were enrolled. These regions represent the majority of migrants in Portugal (Serviço de Estrangeiros e Fronteiras, 2017). For the focus groups with health workers, the research team contacted and invited primary healthcare professionals of Lisbon and the Tagus Valley region, with the support of ARSLVT (Regional Health Administration of Lisbon and the Tagus Valley). Each focus group included individuals of both sexes, from different professional occupations (office workers, nurses and doctors), with different experiences and from services with different proportions of migrant users. A total of six focus groups were formed, one for each group of migrants (African, Brazilian and Eastern European) and professional occupation (office workers, nurses and doctors).

Data Collection Procedure

The organization and conduction of the focus groups are two relevant features to ensure and maximize the quality of the data collected (Côté-Arsenault & Morrison-Beedy, 2005; Goldman & Schmalz, 2001; Hyde et al., 2005; Krueger & Casey, 2000; Morgan, 2001; Patton, 2002).

The focus groups technique enables the collection of data in a fairly short period of time (usually sessions last about 90 minutes). The selection of a friendly and welcoming environment is crucial for the success of this technique. The setting of the focus group should be neutral to the participants, comfortable and inviting to active participation. Focus groups should be conducted in places with adequate acoustic conditions and which ensure privacy. Participants, moderator and co-moderator should be seated in a way that everyone can see each other (e.g., in a circle), as this position promotes group interaction, favours group dynamics and allows for a successful conduction of the discussion.

The role of the moderator is essential for facilitating and encouraging the group discussion in a neutral way which supports free expression of opinion, while keeping the discussion in line with what is planned, refocusing on the topic when necessary and to ensure the greatest quantity and quality of data (Côté-Arsenault & Morrison-Beedy, 2005; Kidd & Parshall, 2000; Morgan, 2001). The main challenge of the moderator is to involve participants so they feel comfortable enough to share with the group what they think and feel about a particular topic. The moderator should create a context of empathy and know how to promote participants' confidence in themselves, in the process and in the correct use of the results. For this reason, focus groups must be conducted by a team with technical skills and experience (active listening, empathic expression, systematic observation, and with the capacity to waive the influence of their own values and perspectives to the participants).

For the present study, focus groups were conducted in Instituto de Higiene e Medicina Tropical and in immigrant associations (that were project partners), neutral settings that provided a comfortable and welcoming environment. Each discussion session lasted around one hour and a half and were conducted in Portuguese. A moderator and a co-moderator with expertise in focus groups technique conducted all the group discussions.

At the beginning of each discussion session, information was presented about the study objectives and purpose, how the session would be conducted and the procedure of data collection. Each session was audio-taped in order to optimize data collection and facilitate the transcription of group discussions for analysis. Informed, written and voluntary consent was obtained from each participant, safeguarding his/her anonymity and the confidentiality of data. The study was approved by the Ethical Committee of the Institute of Hygiene and Tropical Medicine, New University of Lisbon.

Instrument

Two guides were elaborated, one for the groups of immigrants and another for the groups of health workers. These guides did not have the purpose of imposing a rigid structure, but rather orienting the discussions around the defined themes, allowing the organization of data collection. In both immigrants and health workers' groups, the sessions explored participants' perceptions about barriers in migrants' access and utilization of health services and suggestions to promote access and utilization of health services by migrants.

Data Analysis

All discussions were transcribed, and transcripts were verified through audiotape recordings for accuracy. Data were analysed according to the content analysis procedure commonly used in qualitative methodology (Bardin, 2004; Krueger & Casey, 2000; Morgan, 2001). Content analysis is built from the participants' concrete reality and their history, and takes place in three phases: pre-analysis, in which the empirical material is organized in order to systematize the initial ideas and to create the categories of analysis; the exploration of the material, in which after the definition of the categories of analysis the empirical material is organized; and the treatment of the results obtained and their interpretation. In this way, the theoretical questions previously defined in this study were analysed together with the general topics of the discussions, in order to elaborate the first items for analysis. The analysis began by reading through the transcripts and listening to the audio records in order to identify the relevant ideas and concepts emerging in the group sessions. Subsequently, on the basis of the thematic topics, initial categories were created that later evolved and changed during the analysis. Afterward, two independent investigators coded and organized data according to these categories. The opinions of participants on the different topics were analysed taking into account the group agreements and individual contributions. The different responses were grouped into discursive categories taking into account how regularly certain thematic elements appeared and repeated in the discussions. Coded transcripts were reviewed, and overall there was high agreement between researchers. In the few cases where agreement was not achieved, a discussion was held between investigators to resolve inconsistencies of interpretation. Firstly, the analyses focused on each focus group separately and then on the comparison between groups. To maintain participants' confidentiality, names of individuals and institutions were not included in transcripts, and all participants are referred to as either women or participants in this chapter. Quotes were chosen to best illustrate the themes that emerged from data analysis.

RESULTS

Focus Groups with Immigrants

Migrants' Perceptions of Factors Influencing Access and Utilization of Health Services

Migrant participants highlighted positive factors that facilitate migrants' utilization of health services, namely their trust in the health workers (*"I think the whole community has a great trust in the doctors"* [African]), as well as the presence of health workers from their country of origin (*"We talk to them and they provide more response than the others"* [Eastern European]). However, participants also identified barriers that hinder access and utilization of health services, namely related to economic, legal, linguistic, relational, cultural and structural factors.

Some African and Brazilian participants pointed out economic difficulties, often experienced by migrants, as a barrier: *"(...) when they try to gain access they are not able to do that, because they cannot afford it"* [Brazilian]. In addition, in African participants' opinion, being undocumented is a key factor hindering access to health services: *"When one is undocumented and gets sick, [he] doesn't have a right to health services"* [African]. According to some participants, migrants often do not know or do not understand the legislation regulating their access to health services and the procedures needed to get access: *"(...) they don't have minimal information (...) they don't even know they have the right to the medical card, even when they make social security contributions"* [Brazilian]. In this context, some African participants reported that undocumented migrants may use alternative strategies to obtain healthcare. It was also reported that some migrants may use hospital services more due to the barriers faced when seeking healthcare in primary care services.

Communication constraints due to linguistic differences between patients and health workers also were reported by African and Eastern European migrants, stating that often migrants have difficulties in expressing themselves (*"Sometimes they [migrants] want to communicate or present the situation but they are not able to do that, and sometimes that makes them angry (...) technicians don't understand them"* [African]), and in understanding what the professionals tell them (*"[the doctor] speaks fast"* [Eastern European]). Another issue mentioned was the "passive" attitude that migrants often have towards the health services: *"People meet a person with a lighter skin tone, speaking in an austere way, and that blocks them"* [African]. Also, it was referred that some migrants may experience stressful situations when accessing the services: *"(...) when they get there, they are already nervous because they couldn't solve other personal matters, and then the administrative staff has to deal with that irritability"* [African].

Participants also mentioned situations in which the relationship with health workers was sometimes difficult due to the attitudes, including arrogance, lack of empathy or unwillingness to help on the part of some professionals: *"some people think (...) 'oh, she comes here, she's pregnant, and she doesn't have to pay anything (...) my sister pays contributions and doesn't have the same privileges', and so they hold back and are not so open to help"* [African]; *"the receptionist (...) is the first contact and generally they are arrogant"* [Brazilian]. Some participants commented that sometimes when patient-health worker interaction was difficult the continuation of health services use was compromised: *"it's something you live once, and then you think three times before you come back"* [Brazilian]. Participants also reported a lack of sensitivity by some health workers due to cultural differences: *"They don't want to understand; they want to impose their own rules. They don't want to understand that there are different cultures, it's that way and nothing more!"* [African]. For some participants, especially Africans, there is lack of information about some cultural and religious practices: *"Nurses decided to make a flyer about eating habits and then they asked me to translate it into creole (...) when I started reading I realized that there was nothing there that we usually eat!"* [African]. In some participants' opinions, health workers sometimes have preconceptions about migrants: *"(...) there is prejudice in society against the migrant"* [Brazilian]. Some participants described how health workers' less positive attitudes may translate into a refusal to provide healthcare. In those circumstances, migrants may feel restricted in their capacity to claim their rights, which contributes to the worsening of their health status. It was also mentioned that some health workers seem unaware of the legislation regulating migrants' access to healthcare: *"(...) sometimes, people have the right to go there, but as the office worker does not know the law and doesn't even care about knowing it, it's just 'look, don't come here, just go to the hospital'"* [African]. In the opinion of African participants, the lack of experience of health professionals in diagnosing and treating tropical diseases can also be a barrier in access to health services: *"Sometimes there are things we have that they have never seen"* [African]. Nevertheless, some participants described positive attitudes from the health workers: *"Many times, they want to help and are able to get around [the barriers]"* [African].

Finally, participants identified barriers related to the health services. Some Brazilian and Eastern European migrants emphasized the overload of bureaucratic procedures: *"(...) I just wanted a blood test but my doctor gave me so many forms to fill... I just didn't go"* [Eastern European]. Some African participants mentioned difficulties in registering as a patient, often in relation to problems in the information system used: *"I believe it is very old"* [African]. Another difficulty reported by participants was the long waiting time for medical appointments, with implications for migrants' health (*"... you have to wait months and months"* [Eastern European]), as well as the schedules of primary health centres that often are incompatible with the demands of professional occupations (*"Most of us choose to work, and not to lose a day's pay"* [Eastern European]). The lack of human resources also can limit services' ability to respond: *"it's too much work for so a few people"* [African]. Nevertheless, a small group of participants stated that migrants' difficulties in accessing health services are similar to those of the general population: *"The problems immigrants face (...) are faced by the Portuguese population"* [Brazilian].

Suggestions to Improve Migrants' Access and Utilization of Health Services

One of the most common suggestions made by migrant participants for the improvement of access and utilization of health services was to capacitate health workers for cultural diversity: *"(...) to provide more training about culture and cultural diversity, about the context"* [African].

Some African participants considered that health workers should know how to communicate in other languages (*"... if the doctor speaks our language, it will be so much easier"* [African]) and suggested the presence of translators in the health services. Migrants also proposed the use of a telephone service to make medical appointments in other languages: *"(...) a call-centre with people speaking different languages"* [Eastern European]. Migrant participants also suggested the integration of alternative or non-conventional medicine in the health services: *"When will the healers be included in the hospitals and primary health centres? There must be a balance between Medicines"* [African].

Some participants stated that the information available about the functioning of health services and the legislation on access to healthcare is insufficient. In this area, they suggested a stronger investment in information and training, both from the side of migrant populations (*"It is important that the population also gets information and training"* [Brazilian]; *"It is really needed an understanding also from the part of the Brazilian who arrives"* [Brazilian]), and from the health workers' side (*"... I think it's key that they [health workers] have access to the correct information, and that comes from the services' directors"* [Brazilian]).

Some African participants referred to the need to create a closer relationship with the community, proposing an investment in community intervention and health education through cooperation with migrant associations, religious communities and schools. Another issue mentioned was the involvement of the immigrant communities in the definition and implementation of action strategies regarding access to health services: *"(...) we would like to also be heard"* [African]. Eastern European participants emphasized the importance of providing household consultations as a way to facilitate access to healthcare: *"(...) the sick person can't get out of the bed"* [Eastern European].

Eastern European participants highlighted the importance of monitoring the functioning of health services: *"(...) for instance, many consultations don't start on time and that increases the waiting time"* [Eastern European]. Also, some Brazilian participants highlighted the need to create sanctions if the health workers do not comply with migrants' legal rights to access health services.

Finally, participants emphasized the need to diminish bureaucratic procedures in the access to health services as a way to promote their use, and other participants reported the need to update the information system: *"(...) I believe they have to update it, the reality has changed"* [African].

Focus Groups with Health Workers

Perceptions about Factors Influencing Migrants' Access and Utilization of Health Services

Health workers pointed out various barriers - economic, knowledge-based, linguistic, cultural, relational and structural - which hinder migrants' access and use of health services.

One reported barrier was the socioeconomic difficulties of immigrants, which sometimes results in the inability to afford healthcare expenses. Some health workers mentioned that migrants did not seem to know their rights (*"... [Brazilian] women used to go to the doctor only in the last semester of their pregnancies. Why? Because they didn't know they had the right to be consulted throughout pregnancy"* [Nurse]), as well as about the procedures needed to access the services (*"not everybody knows the type of documents they have to bring"* [Office worker]). The nurses' focus group emphasized that migrants are not fully informed about the structure and functioning of health services, nor the different available services, which leads to a reduced utilization of health services, particularly in the field of preventative medicine: *"There are a lot of migrants who don't know that there is maternal-infant surveillance (...)"* [Nurse]. On the other hand, according to participants, some health workers also lack knowledge about the legal rights to healthcare: *"I don't know how to answer to certain questions, maybe because there is no law, or because I don't have knowledge about it"* [Office worker]. In participants' opinion, this can hinder the patient's registration in the National Health System, and lead to undue user charges: *"There are some places where healthcare fees are incorrectly charged to new-born children"* [Nurse]. Health workers also stated that they are not aware of the available services for specialized care for patients, for example with economic difficulties (*"We don't know where to send them"* [Office worker]) and the available resources in the field of intercultural mediation (*"I didn't even know there were cultural mediators"* [Doctor]). Health workers' lack of practice in diagnosing and treating tropical or other unusual diseases was also referred to as an obstacle to the clinical practice (*"Pathologies can go unnoticed and sometimes we are not very sure about what we are doing"* [Doctor]). Nurses in particular revealed their unawareness of the vaccination programs in the countries of origin and the difficulty felt to apply the national vaccination plan.

Several health workers emphasized difficulties in communication due to linguistic differences between health workers and migrant patients: *"(...) neither in Portuguese, neither in English. She [the patient] only speaks her own dialect, and so it is really difficult to communicate"* [Office worker]. Particularly some doctors reported difficulties in communication due to the complexity of the medical terminology. Office workers described that, sometimes, in this context, some doctors refuse to conduct the consultation in other languages: *"I know that some doctors won't speak English, so migrants will leave just as they arrived"* [Office worker].

Some health workers considered that cultural and religious practices are factors influencing the use of health services. Especially, different notions of health and illness were reported by some doctors and nurses as potentially hindering migrants' use of health services: *"It has to do with the way they understand pathologies, the diagnosis..."* [Doctor]. According to some participants, gender roles also hamper the provision of healthcare: *"There are some groups in which females can't go to an appointment with a male doctor"* [Office worker]. Some professionals reported that the patterns of healthcare use in the country of origin impact the perception of need of using the health services in Portugal: *"Many times people have the primary healthcare centre near (...), but for them it is not important because in Africa kids go years without seeing a doctor"* [Nurse]. Migrants' expectations toward healthcare in the host country were mentioned by some health workers as an important issue that may foment dissatisfaction and act as a barrier to the continuity of health care. In addition, participants pointed to health workers' lack of knowledge of cultural and religious practices as a factor that potentially influences healthcare provision and the quality of diagnosis (*"They have several things related to mysticism and religion that may confound our assessment"* [Nurse]). Notwithstanding, for some health workers, cultural issues do not influence migrants' healthcare seeking (*"Beliefs don't interfere in anything. They go [to the doctor] anyway"* [Doctor]).

Several participants pointed out difficulties in the professional-patient relationship which, in their opinion, are connected to the lack of sensitivity to cultural differences: *"From a cultural point of view there are some difficulties in understanding, in wanting to understand, in finding solutions to overcome difficulties"* [Doctor]. Some health workers admitted having heard about a few episodes of discrimination and prejudice from some professionals.

Health workers also mentioned barriers to migrants' access and utilization related to services. The lack of human resources was reported across all three groups of professionals: *"Nowadays, with restrained expenses, (...) we have human resources at minimal limits, maybe even less"* [Doctor]. According to participants, these circumstances restrict their time and capacity to respond to migrants' needs: *"(...) when we are alone in the maternal health consultation, for instance, and we have 20 people in the waiting room..."* [Nurse]. The reduced schedules of primary care centres restrict migrants' access to healthcare, according to participants, and especially nurses: *"There are several [services] closing at 18.00, others are closed during weekends, closed during holidays"* [Nurse]. Some nurses outlined the difficulty of migrants to make use of services, particularly due to the limited hours of the primary care centres: *"(...) if a migrant misses work (...), his contract won't be renewed. If the contract is not renewed, the residence permit won't be renewed"* [Nurse]. Some nurses and doctors reported the overload of bureaucratic procedures as a factor that often hinders migrants' utilization of health services: *"Primary healthcare centres are an intense bureaucracy for migrants"* [Doctor]. Another obstacle is, according to the participants, the ambiguity of legislation about the registration of undocumented immigrants: *"The legislation is ambiguous and the application of the law allows everything and anything, even for those who understand it"* [Nurse]. Some nurses and office workers also reported difficulties in the registration of patients due to the complexity of the information system: *"The software is old, outdated and complicated"* [Office worker].

Suggestions to Improve Migrants' Access and Utilization of Health Services

The discourses of some health workers revealed the need to comply with legislation about access to health services (*"... it's not sufficient to just put in on paper (...), people have to comply with it and that's the problem"* [Nurse]), and to standardize the procedures along the different health centres of the National Health Service. Health workers suggested ways to improve their knowledge about legislation regulating access to health services and associated procedures, for instance through the implementation of training oriented for all professional groups: *"... Let's not only talk about training for technical assistants and nurses. I believe that even the executive directors must have knowledge about the legislation"* [Nurse]. Office workers were unanimous in pointing out the need for training about the health information software system, given the difficulties they felt when registering patients: *"to prevent us from incurring injustices"* [Office worker]. A nurse highlighted that a mapping of the existing community services should be developed, allowing for better articulation between community resources and health services: *"(...) to understand the available community resources, and which partnerships can be established..."* [Nurse].

Another suggestion was to improve health workers' competencies for dealing with heterogeneous migrant populations, through cultural diversity training: *"It wouldn't be a bad idea to start organizing workshops about this issue (...) from the assistant to the doctor (...) but it has to be mandatory, otherwise no one will go"* [Doctor]. Some doctors suggested the involvement of the community in the implementation of these training actions. Training on other languages and tropical diseases was also highlighted (*"It would be really important that primary health centres provided training [in other languages]"* [Office worker]; *"(...) tropical diseases are not so easy to diagnose"* [Doctor]). Another topic was the need to put into practice the communication competencies acquired during technical training: *"Maybe we should remember the importance of communication when we are caring for the patients"* [Nurse].

Health workers also stressed the need to promote health education in migrant communities, as a way to improve migrants' health: *"(...) to increase awareness for health issues (...) and to tell them 'you go to the health centre for this and for that'"* [Doctor]. Several doctors proposed the development of informative brochures translated into several languages about infant health, as well as about migrants' legal rights and functioning of health services.

Some discourses reinforced the relevance of creating a proximity relationship through community intervention. Particularly, doctors emphasized this need regarding preventative care: *"to intervene in the community (...) preventative care is not even an issue"* [Doctor]. The intercultural mediator was acknowledged as an important figure in the resolution of several problems and in follow-up migrant patients. Office workers suggested that migrants study Portuguese to help overcome linguistic barriers.

Finally, participants made some suggestions about the structure and organization of healthcare services, highlighting the need for cooperation between different health workers to improve provision of healthcare (*"... even we need someone to help us solving the questions they present us at the desk"* [Office worker]). They also suggested the creation of multidisciplinary teams for implementing integrated responses to migrants' problems. Some nurses and office workers pointed out that the increase of human resources should be made a priority.

CONCLUSION

This study using focus groups has provided in-depth insights into the multiple factors related to barriers in migrants' access and utilization of health services, as expressed by both migrants and health workers. Overall, participants reported that migrants' use of health services is often influenced by factors at individual, health workers and health services levels. In the overall analysis, individual factors were the most frequently mentioned by participants.

The disadvantaged socioeconomic conditions and job insecurity may limit migrants' ability to access services and bear the costs of healthcare. In addition, as mentioned by some participants, in a context of social vulnerability, health is not considered a priority, which reduces the adoption of preventive practices. These results suggest that potential difficulties in the migration process may have repercussions on the health status of these populations, as mentioned by other authors (Judge et al., 2006; Norredam, Nielsen & Krasnik, 2010). Even though current legal framework establishes access to health care for all, it was reported that in some cases the undocumented status was a barrier. The lack of knowledge of both migrants and professionals about migrants' current legal rights has been consistently pointed out as a factor impacting law enforcement. As a result, some undocumented migrants may use services mainly in an emergency situation. This finding corroborates previous studies (Dias & Gonçalves, 2007; Ingleby et al., 2005). These data reinforce the relevance of developing strategies to improve the knowledge of all stakeholders about migrants' rights to healthcare, contributing to a greater and more adequate use of services, especially by the most vulnerable groups (Ingleby et al., 2005, Manfellotto, 2002).

Other factors influencing migrants' access and use of health services are related to the interaction between health workers and migrants. Difficulties in communication due to linguistic differences were expressed by several participants from both groups. In fact, language barriers hinder the sharing of information and the expression of health needs by immigrants, as well as the professionals' performance, especially regarding diagnosis and treatment (Fonseca et al., 2007; Hultsjö & Hjelm, 2005; Scheppers et al., 2006). Professionals' limited social and cultural skills, accentuated by their insufficient knowledge of the cultural and religious practices of migrant communities, were also considered a barrier by both migrants and health workers. Participants stated that such gaps may impact the relationship that the health professional establishes with the migrant patient, as well as the clinical practice itself (Esteva et al., 2006; Scheppers et al., 2006). The difficulty in the diagnosis and treatment of tropical diseases has also been described as a barrier in the provision of healthcare and as an obstacle to the migrants' continued use of health services, which has been mentioned in previous studies (Esteva et al., 2006; Vázquez-Villegas, 2006). A few episodes of discrimination by health workers were described during the focus groups. It was emphasized that their perception of health problems is sometimes an expression of the prejudices and stereotypes attributed to certain groups of migrants, which can lead to situations of discrimination and stigmatization in the healthcare context. The literature has shown that stereotypes, prejudices and negative attitudes are determinants in the quality of professional-patient interaction, which may result in users' dissatisfaction or non-use of services (Fuertes & Martín Laso, 2006; Ingleby et al., 2005). Future research should explore healthcare professionals' attitudes towards migrant populations taking into account the sociodemographic characteristics of the patients, and the impact on the quality of the care provided.

Participants agreed upon several aspects of the functioning of the health services limiting their use, such as the lack of human resources, inconvenient schedules and excessive bureaucratic procedures. The functioning and organization of health services restrain access and use by the general population. However, these difficulties tend to affect immigrants more, since they often find themselves impacted by administrative problems, precarious labour situations with excessive workloads and little social protection (Dias, Severo & Barros, 2008; Dias & Rocha, 2009; Fennelly, 2006).

In general, there were differences among subgroups of participants regarding the way they perceive factors influencing access and use of services. In the migrants' group, African participants reported more often the lack of economic resources as an obstacle to the use of services, which may be related in part to a potential worse socioeconomic situation of this group. Eastern and African participants more frequently reported barriers related to the expression of symptoms and recognition of disease. These results point out that cultural issues influence the way in which the symptoms are recognized and expressed by migrants and potentially the way they are understood by professionals (Anderson et al., 2003). In addition, African and Eastern European participants mentioned the lack of translators or interpreters in health services as an important barrier.

In the health workers' group, differences were found mainly between office workers and doctors/nurses regarding their perceptions of the factors of access and use of services. In fact, these topics were explored in focus groups differently: office workers emphasized issues related to the procedures of access to healthcare, whereas doctors and nurses emphasized professionals' unawareness of cultural and religious practices and its influence in care provision. In addition, nurses differed from doctors and office workers in terms of the importance attributed to the social and cultural competencies of health workers. These results seem to suggest that nurses may be more sensitized and aware of these issues than the other professional groups. These discrepancies are likely to reflect the different roles that these groups play and the type of contact they have with migrant patients, which reinforces the need to develop training tailored to various professionals.

The perceptions of migrants and health workers about the barriers to migrants' access and use of services reinforce the existence of opportunities for intervention. Indeed, both groups of participants presented a set of proposals and recommendations focused on the adequacy of health services to culturally diverse populations, and the promotion of access and utilization of health services by migrants.

The use of the focus group technique in health research has several advantages. One of the advantages of this technique relates to the interaction between the participants (Kidd & Parshall, 2000; Warr, 2005). This interaction allows the researcher/ moderator to analyse how the person constructs his own reality, and to interpret the participants' views as if in a social network (Green & Thorogood, 2004). This interactive nature is also useful in the sense that disagreements and contradictions occur and lead participants to develop their own views and to critically analyse their own opinions as well as those of the other participants (Krueger & Casey, 2000). On the other hand, group dynamics may lead participants to get involved in the discussion, and to share their answers and comments with the group and not only with the researcher. This may overcome the barriers between participants and the moderator and remove the defensive attitudes that some questions may generate (Hyde et al., 2005). In this study, this was the case, for example, with the discussion of how migrants' undocumented status impacted access and utilization of health services; some participants reported episodes of care refusal and situations of discrimination.

The focus group technique may provide access to the language and the cognitive, emotional and social models of the participants, as well as to the production of the meanings, perceptions, attitudes and actions (Hyde et al., 2005; Morgan, 2001). In this technique, participants are not only the subject of study but also donors of information (Krueger & Casey, 2000). The priorities of a focus group are what participants consider most important and the discussion is guided by their interests. When a focus group is conducted well, participants work in parallel with the researcher, leading the discussion in new and unexpected directions. Group dynamics may activate responses and provide awareness about connected experiences and beliefs, allowing the emergence of questions not anticipated by the researchers. This does not happen when the discussion is strictly guided by the hypotheses and interpretations of the research (Rich & Ginsburg, 1999).

Due to the inherent nature and characteristics of the focus group technique and the participants' selection process, the views and perceptions expressed in the group discussions cannot represent those of the study populations. However, the findings corroborate the conclusions of other studies on migrants' access and utilization of health services. The group interaction may influence data collection in two different ways. On one hand, focus groups tend to facilitate openness and exchange of personal experiences, and participants feel more comfortable expressing their opinion in a group than privately (Morgan, 2001; Zwane, Mngadi & Nxumalo, 2004). On the other hand, interaction may be one of the limitations of this technique, in the sense that the group dynamics influence strongly the individual contributions. Being in a group may lead participants to feel constrained or inhibited to talk about personal or "confidential" information, and to silence opinions conflicting with the majority of the group given the personal exposure of this technique. Another of the limitations is that the participants' responses may be more likely to result from a bias derived from the pressure to conform to the norms of the group or from a need to self-present themselves in a socially desirable way. Nevertheless, health and migration are potentially sensitive issues, and several studies have proposed that focus groups are a proper method to approach such sensitive topics (Farquhar & Das, 1999; Hyde et al., 2005; Ingham, Vanwesenbeeck & Kirkland, 1999). Focus groups promote a relatively spontaneous relationship between the participants and a context of some intimacy, and therefore may give the participants the opportunity to talk about sensitive topics with less inhibitions. On the other hand, participants may provide support in the expression of feelings and common experiences, and often uninhibited participants encourage shy participants to share their ideas (Kitzinger, 2000).

In order to maximize the potentialities of a qualitative data collection technique such as focus groups, particular attention must be given to the study protocol, planning and procedures. Especially, the attitude of the moderator greatly influences the quality of the information obtained in the group discussions. The moderator must be trained to reduce his influence in terms of expectations, naturally welcoming the different opinions without conflict or trying to influence. The discussion should not be overly rigid, and it is important that it responds to the dynamics and priorities of each group, while also exploring in depth the research question (Kitzinger, 2000). In this sense, the role of the moderator is extremely relevant when sensitive issues are approached (Farquhar & Das, 1999).

Globally, the use of focus groups in this study contributed to produce rich, relevant and useful knowledge potentially translatable into good practices for the promotion of access and use of health services among a most vulnerable population like migrants. In an innovative way, through focus groups the study involved migrants and health workers as relevant and active stakeholders in knowledge production and recommendation of proposals to improve migrants' access to health services. This created an opportunity for enhancing the empowerment of migrant communities to advocate for their health rights. Indeed, active participation and empowerment were transversal guiding principles during group discussions and were essential for the promotion of capacity-building of migrant communities towards their health protection and promotion, contributing to a social innovation process. During this process, it was possible to: promote a relationship of trust with migrants and with health workers; to increase relevance of the main questions around migrants' access and utilization of health services and identify new questions prioritized by communities, allowing an increased knowledge that translates communities' needs; raise awareness of both migrant and health workers communities about the topics explored; and strengthen the sense of domain, regulation and co-responsibility in contributing to improve migrants' access to health services.

The focus groups approach represents an important contribution for better understanding the perspectives and experiences of migrant communities regarding their health, for interpreting the findings in a contextualized way and potentially using them through effective health actions that address migrants' needs. A remaining challenge is to develop strategies and mechanisms to assess the impact of the focus group technique in studies with different dimensions, contexts and populations and understand the dynamic changes it can produce in terms of community participation, capacity building and empowerment.

REFERENCES

Anderson, L.M., Scrimshaw, S.C., Fullilove, M.T., Fielding, J.E., Normand, J., & Task Force on Community Preventive Services (2003). Culturally competent healthcare systems: a systematic review. *American Journal of Preventive Medicine, 24* (3), 68-79.

Barbour, R., & Kitzinger, J. (1999). *Developing focus group research: Politics, theory and practice.* London: SAGE Publications Ltd.

Bardin, L. (2004). *Análise de conteúdo* [Content analysis] (3rd ed.). Lisboa: Edições 70, Lda.

Blair, A., & Schneeberg, A. (2014). Changes in the 'healthy migrant effect' in Canada: Are recent immigrants healthier than they were a decade ago? *Journal of Immigrant and Minority Health, 16* (1), 136-142.

Bowen, G. (2008). Naturalistic inquiry and the saturation concept: a research note. *Qualitative Research, 8* (1), 137-152.

Buja, A., Fusco, M., Furlan, P., Bertoncello, C., Baldovin, T., & Casale, P. et al. (2013). Characteristics, processes, management and outcome of accesses to accident and emergency departments by citizenship. *International Journal of Public Health, 59* (1), 167-174.

Côté-Arsenault, D., & Morrison-Beedy, D. (2005). Maintaining your focus in focus groups: Avoiding common mistakes. *Research in Nursing & Health, 28* (2), 172-179.

Davies, A., Basten, A., & Frattini, C. (2006). *Migration: a social determinant of the health of migrants (Background paper)*. Geneva: IOM Migration Health Department.

Dias, S., & Gonçalves, A. (2007). Migração e saúde [Migration and health]. *Migrações, 1*, 15-26.

Dias, S., & Rocha, C. (2009). *Saúde sexual e reprodutiva de mulheres imigrantes africanas e brasileiras: um estudo qualitativo*. Lisboa: Alto-Comissariado para a Imigração e Diálogo Intercultural [Sexual and reproductive health of African and Brazilian immigrant women: a qualitative study. Lisbon: High Commission for Immigration and Intercultural Dialogue].

Dias, S., Gama, A., Cortes, M., & de Sousa, B. (2011a). Healthcare-seeking patterns among immigrants in Portugal. *Health & Social Care in the Community, 19* (5), 514-521.

Dias, S., Gama, A., Silva, A., Cargaleiro, H., & O. Martins, M. (2011b). [Barriers in access and utilization of health services among immigrants: the perspective of health professionals]. *Acta Médica Portuguesa, 24* (4), 511-516.

Dias, S., Matos, M., & Gonçalves, A. (2001). Comportamento sexual – auto-relatos numa comunidade migrante. *Revista Portuguesa de Pedagogia,* [Sexual behavior - self-reports in a migrant community. Portuguese Journal of Pedagogy] *35* (2), 137-153.

Dias, S., Matos, M., & Gonçalves, A. (2002). Conhecimentos, atitudes e comportamentos face ao VIH numa comunidade migrante – implicações para a intervenção. *Psicologia, Saúde & Doença*, [Knowledge, attitudes and behavior towards HIV in a migrant community - implications for the intervention. Psychology, Health & Sickness] *3* (1), 89-102.

Dias, S., Severo, M., & Barros, H. (2008). Determinants of health care utilization by immigrants in Portugal. *BMC Health Services Research, 8*, 207.

Esteva, M., Cabrera, S., Remartinez, D., Díaz, A., & March, S. (2006). [Perception of difficulties in family medicine in the delivery of health to economic immigrants]. *Atención Primaria, 37* (3), 154-159.

Eurostat (2017, August 29). *Migration and migrant population statistics - Statistics Explained.* Retrieved from http://ec.europa.eu/eurostat/statistics-explained/index.php/Migration_and_migrant_population_statistics

Farquhar, C., & Das, R. (1999). Are focus groups suitable for 'sensitive' topics? In R. Barbour & J. Kitzinger, *Developing focus group research: Politics, theory and practice* (pp. 47-63). London: SAGE Publications Ltd.

Fennelly, K. (2006). Listening to the experts: provider recommendations on the health needs of immigrants and refugees. *Journal of Cultural Diversity, 13* (4), 190-201.

Fern, E. (2001). *Advanced Focus Group Research*. Thousand Oaks: SAGE Publications, Inc.

Fonseca, M., Esteves, A., McGarrigle, J., & Silva, S. (2007). Saúde e integração dos imigrantes em Portugal: uma perspectiva geográfica e política [Health and integration of immigrants in Portugal: A geographical and political perspective]. *Migrações, 1*, 27-52.

Frith, H. (2000). Focusing on sex: using focus groups in sex research. *Sexualities, 3* (3), 275-297.

Fuertes, C., & Martín Laso, M. (2006). The immigrant in primary care consultations. *Anales Del Sistema Sanitario De Navarra, 29* (Supl. 1), 9-25.

Giannoni, M., Franzini, L., & Masiero, G. (2016). Migrant integration policies and health inequalities in Europe. *BMC Public Health, 16*, 1-14.

Goddard, M., & Smith, P. (2001). Equity of access to health care services: Theory and evidence from the UK. *Social Science & Medicine, 53*(9), 1149-1162.

Goldman, K. & Schmalz, K. (2001). Focus on Focus Groups! *Health Promotion Practice, 2* (1): 14-19.

Graetz, V., Rechel, B., Groot, W., Norredam, M., & Pavlova, M. (2017). Utilization of health care services by migrants in Europe—a systematic literature review. *British Medical Bulletin, 121* (1), 5-18.

Green, J., & Thorogood, N. (2004). *Qualitative methods for health research.* London: SAGE Publications Ltd.

Halcomb, E., Gholizadeh, L., DiGiacomo, M., Phillips, J., & Davidson, P. (2007). Literature review: considerations in undertaking focus group research with culturally and linguistically diverse groups. *Journal of Clinical Nursing, 16* (6), 1000-1011.

Hargreaves, S., Friedland, J., Gothard, P., Saxena, S., Millington, H., & Eliahoo, J. et al. (2006). Impact on and use of health services by international migrants: questionnaire survey of inner city London A&E attenders. *BMC Health Services Research, 6*, 1-7.

Hollander, J. (2004). The Social Contexts of Focus Groups. *Journal of Contemporary Ethnography, 33* (5), 602-637.

Houghton, C., Casey, D., Shaw, D., & Murphy, K. (2013). Rigour in qualitative case-study research. *Nurse Researcher, 20* (4), 12-17.

Hultsjö, S., & Hjelm, K. (2005). Immigrants in emergency care: Swedish health care staff's experiences. *International Nursing Review, 52* (4), 276-285.

Hyde, A., Howlett, E., Brady, D., & Drennan, J. (2005). The focus group method: Insights from focus group interviews on sexual health with adolescents. *Social Science & Medicine, 61* (12), 2588-2599.

Ingham, R., Vanwesenbeeck, I., & Kirkland, D. (1999). Interviewing on sensitive topics. In A.A. Memon & R. Bull (Eds.), *Handbook of the Psychology of Interviewing* (pp. 145-164), Michigan: John Wiley & Sons Ltd.

Ingleby, D., Chimienti, M., Hatziprokopiou, P., Ormond, M., & Freitas C. (2005). The role of health in integration. In M.L. Fonseca & J. Malheiros

(Coord.), *Social integration and mobility: education, housing & health* (pp. 101-137). Lisboa: Centro de Estudos Geográficos: Estudos para o Planeamento Regional e Urbano [Center for Geographical Studies: Studies for Regional and Urban Planning].

International Organization for Migration (2004). *Glossary on migration.* Geneva: IOM.

Judge, K., Platt, S., Costongs, C., & Jurczak, K. (2006). *Health inequalities: a challenge for Europe. Discussion paper.* London: UK Presidency of the EU.

Kidd, P., & Parshall, M. (2000). Getting the focus and the group: Enhancing analytical rigor in focus group research. *Qualitative Health Research, 10* (3), 293-308.

Kitzinger, J. (2000). Focus groups. In C. Pope & N. Mays (Eds.), *Qualitative research in health care* (2nd ed) (pp. 21-31). London: British Medical Association.

Kristiansen, M., Mygind, A., & Krasnik, A. (2007). Health effects of migration. *Danish Medical Bulletin, 54* (1), 46-47.

Krueger, R. & Casey, M. (2000). *Focus groups: A practical guide for applied research* (3rd ed.). Thousand Oaks, CA: Sage Publications.

Kuerban, A. (2016). Healthy migrant effect on smoking behavior among Asian immigrants in the United States. *Journal of Immigrant and Minority Health, 18* (1), 94-101.

Lester, H., Tritter, J.Q., Sorohan, H. (2005). Patients' and health professionals' views on primary care for people with serious mental illness: focus group study. *BMJ, 330* (7500), 1122.

Linhorst, D.M. (2002). A review of the use and potential of focus groups in social work research. *Qualitative Social Work, 1* (2), 208-228.

Lobdell, D.T., Gilboa, S., Mendola, P., & Hesse, B.W. (2005). Use of focus groups for the environmental health researcher. *Journal of Environmental Health, 67* (9), 36-42.

Machado, M.C., Santana, P., Carreiro, M., Nogueira, H., Barroso, M., & Dias, A. (2006). *Iguais ou diferentes? Cuidados de Saúde materno-infantil a uma população de imigrantes* [Equal or different? Maternal and child health care for an immigrant population]. Lisboa: Bial.

Manfellotto, D. (2002). *Case Study 5: From Misinformation and Ignorance to Recognition and Care: Immigrants and Homeless in Rome, Italy in Health Systems Confront Poverty*. Geneva: WHO Regional Office for Europe.

Morgan, D. (2001). Focus Group Interviewing. In J.F. Gubrium & J.A. Holstein (Eds). *Handbook of interview research: context and method.* Thousand Oaks, CA: Sage Publications.

Muennig, P. & Fahs, M.C. (2002). Health status and hospital utilization of recent immigrants to New York City. *Preventive Medicine, 35* (3), 225-231.

Nielsen, S.S. & Krasnik, A. (2010). Poorer self-perceived health among migrants and ethnic minorities versus the majority population in Europe: a systematic review. *International Journal of Public Health, 55*(5), 357–371.

Nordhaus, W.D. (2002). *The health of nations: the contribution of improved health to living standards (Working Paper 8818)*. Retrieved from: http://www.econ.yale.edu/~nordhaus/homepage/health_nber_w8818.pdf.

Norredam, M., Nielsen, S.S., & Krasnik, A. (2010). Migrants' utilization of somatic healthcare services in Europe – a systematic review. *European Journal of Public Health, 20* (5), 555-563.

O'Reilly, M., & Parker, N. (2012). 'Unsatisfactory Saturation': A critical exploration of the notion of saturated sample sizes in qualitative research. *Qualitative Research, 13* (2), 190-197.

Parker, R., Easton, D. & Klein, C.H. (2000). Structural barriers and facilitators in HIV prevention: a review of international research. *AIDS, 14* (Suppl 1), S22-32.

Patton, M. (2002). *Qualitative research and evaluation methods* (3rd ed.). Thousand Oaks, CA: Sage Publications.

Peiro, M.J., & Benedict, R. (2009). *Migration health: better health for all in Europe*. Brussels: International Organization for Migration.

Peterson-Sweeney, K. (2005). The use of focus groups in pediatric and adolescent research. *Journal of Pediatric Health Care, 19* (2), 104-110.

Politzer, R., Yoon, J., Hughes, R., Regan, J., & Gaston, M. (2001). Inequality in America: the contribution of health centers in reducing and eliminating disparities in access to care. *Medical Care Research and Review, 58* (2), 234-248.

Quan, H., Fong, A., De Coster, C., Wang, J., Musto, R., Noseworthy, T.W., & Ghali, W.A. (2006). Variation in health services utilization among ethnic populations. *Canadian Medical Association Journal, 174*, 787-791.

Rechel, B., Mladovsky, P., Ingleby, D., Mackenbach, J.P., McKee, M. (2013). Migration and health in an increasingly diverse Europe. *Lancet, 381* (9873), 1235-1245.

Rich, M., & Ginsburg, K.R. (1999). The reason and rhyme of qualitative research: why, when, and how to use qualitative methods in the study of adolescent health. *Journal of Adolescent Health, 25* (6), 371-378.

Scheppers, E., van Dongen, E., Dekker, J., Geertzen, J. & Dekker, J. (2006). Potential barriers to the use of health services among ethnic minorities: a review. *Family Practice, 23* (3), 325-348.

Serviço de Estrangeiros e Fronteiras (2017). *Relatório de Imigração, Fronteiras e Asilo* [Immigration, Borders and Asylum Report] *2016.* Lisboa: SEF/GEPF.

Simões, J.A.A., Augusto, G.F., Fronteira, I., Hernández-Quevedo C. (2017). Portugal: Health system review. *Health Systems in Transition, 19* (2); 1-184.

Solar, O., & Irwin, A. (2007). *A conceptual framework for action on the social determinants of health. Discussion paper for the Commission on Social Determinants of Health.* Geneva: World Health Organization.

Vázquez-Villegas, J. (2006). [Immigration and Health: a new model of primary care for a new model of society?]. *Atención Primaria, 37*(5), 249-250.

Warr, D. (2005). “It was fun… but we don’t usually talk about these things”: Analyzing sociable interaction in focus groups. *Qualitative Inquiry, 11*(2): 200-225.

World Health Organization (1948). *Constitution of the World Health Organization.* Geneva: WHO.

World Health Organization (2007). *Everybody business: strengthening health systems to improve health outcome: WHO's framework for action*. Geneva: WHO.

World Health Organization (2010). *Health of migrants: the way forward. Report of a Global Consultation, Madrid, Spain, 3-5 March 2010.* Geneva: WHO.

Zwane, I.T., Mngadi, P.T., Nxumalo, M.P. (2004). Adolescents' views on decision-making regarding risky sexual behaviour. *International Nursing Review, 51* (1), 15-22.

In: Advances in Health and Disease. Volume 4 ISBN: 978-1-53613-345-5
Editor: Lowell T. Duncan

Chapter 2

PARVOVIRUS B19 (PVB19) IN PREGNANCY: THE IMPACT OF A PARTIALLY NEGLECTED PROBLEM

Asher Ornoy[1,*] and Zivanit Ergaz[2]
[1]Laboratory of Teratology, Department of Medical Neurobiology, Canada Israel Institute for Medical Research, Hebrew University Hadassah Medical School, Jerusalem, Israel
[2]Department of Neonatology, Hadassah Hebrew University Medical Center, Jerusalem, Israel

ABSTRACT

Parvovirus B19 (PVB19) is a widespread infection that may affects 1-5% of pregnant women; in epidemics, the rate of infection is even higher. In spite of 30%- 50% vertical transmission to the fetus, pregnancy outcome is generally unaffected. Diagnosis of infection is by maternal serology and/or PCR, but fetal infection is diagnosed by PCR from amniotic fluid or, if fetal cordocentesis is carried out, from fetal blood. Reports on major

* Corresponding Author Email: ornoy@cc.huji.ac.il.

congenital anomalies among offspring of mothers infected by Parvovirus B19 affecting different organs are scanty, as the virus does not seem to be a significant human teratogen. However, especially if infection occurs in the first half of pregnancy, it may cause significant fetal damage and rarely also brain anomalies and neurodevelopmental problems. PVB19 is an important cause of fetal loss throughout gestation, especially in the second half of pregnancy; at that time spontaneous fetal loss from other causes is relatively rare. The virus infects fetal erythroid progenitor cells causing apoptosis and, as a result of shortened half-life of erythrocytes moderate to severe fetal anemia. Severe thrombocytopenia is also common. According to its severity, the anemia may lead to high output cardiac failure and therefore non immune hydrops fetalis (NIHF). PVB19 may also directly infect myocardial cells and produce myocarditis that aggravates the cardiac failure. Intrauterine fetal transfusion, which is commonly carried out for the treatment of severe fetal anemia, significantly reduces fetal morbidity. There are little data regarding the long-term neurodevelopmental outcome in infected children. Although data are inadequate, 10-15% of the children infected with PVB19 having hydrops fetalis will suffer from neurodevelopmental impairment. However, there seem to be no data on infected fetuses without hydrops. It is also unknown whether neurodevelopmental sequelae result from the anemia or from the complications of the intrauterine transfusion, since children who had fetal hydrops and intrauterine transfusion due to other etiologies were also found to have a high rate of neurodevelopmental problems. Since PVB19 infection can cause severe morbidity and mortality, it should be part of the routine work up of complicated pregnancies, especially when fetal hydrops is suspected. Risk assessment for maternal infection during pregnancy is particularly important during epidemics when sero-conversion rates are high. Until today, there is no effective immunization against parvovirus.

Keywords: parvovirus B19, pregnancy, non-immune fetal hydrops, anemia, malformations, neurodevelopmental impairment

INTRODUCTION

Parvovirus B19 (PVB19) belongs to the *Parvoviridae* family which has two sub-groups: *Parvovirinae* that infect vertebrates and *Densoviridae* that infect invertebrates. PVB19 belongs to the genus *Erythrovirus* which needs erythroid cells to replicate (Fauquet and Mayo, 2001). Due to its predilection to the erythroid cell line PVB19 infection may result in a destruction of erythropoietic stem cells by the virus, sometimes accompanied by thrombocytopenia (Bonvicini et al., 2011). Hence, infection during pregnancy can often cause severe fetal anemia, high cardiac output failure, non-immune hydrops fetalis (NIHF) and fetal death. Additionally, a variety of symptoms of fetal damage were reported. However, in some of them the causal relationship between the infection and the fetal damage has not been definitely established.

EPIDEMIOLOGY

Most women at child bearing age are already immune to PVB19 having anti PVB19 IgG antibodies in their blood. A current infection is diagnosed either by IgM or by viral DNA analysis in maternal blood.

Evidence for past infection among pregnant women by measuring levels of anti-PVB19 IgG in maternal serums varied between 24% in an Italian population (Di Domenico et al., 2002) to 84% in a Brazilian population (Barros De Freitas et al., 1999). In developing countries the rate is similar. For example, in Sudan, PVB19 IgG antibodies were found in 61.4% of pregnant women, with a higher prevalence in multigravida women (Adam et al., 2015).

The peak incidence of PVB19 infection is in late winter and early spring. The virus is spread by respiratory droplets (Anderson, 1987; Anderson and Cohen, 1987) by blood products, especially pooled factor XIII and IX concentrates (Jordan et al., 1998) and can be transmitted trans-placentally during pregnancy.

Only women who are sero-negative are at risk of acquiring PVB19 infection. An annual sero-conversion of 1.5% among women at childbearing age was described and was unrelated to their occupation and number of young children at home (Koch and Adler, 1989).The risk of infection during pregnancy varies, ranging in endemic areas from about 1% (Baschat et al., 2003), (Tolfvenstam et al., 2001) with the highest rate being 16.5% (Makhseed et al., 1999). Most pregnancies had normal outcome (Di Domenico et al., 2002), (Barros De Freitas et al., 1999), (Gratacos et al.,

1995), (Friese et al., 1991). Seroconversion and vertical transfer are more prevalent during epidemics (Valeur-Jensen et al., 1999) (Gilarranz et al., 2016). The sero-conversion rate was described between 3% (Kerr et al., 1994) to 13.5% (Jensen et al., 2000); the highest rate being 34% (Woernle et al., 1987). The risk of acute infection in pregnancy was found to be in direct correlation with the number of children at home (Valeur-Jensen et al., 1999).

TIMING OF INFECTION DURING PREGNANCY AND FETAL RISK

Maternal infection is generally asymptomatic (Gilarranz et al., 2016) and the risk for fetal damage is low, being only 1-2%; the long-term sequelae is apparently even lower (De Jong et al., 2012). Vertical trans-placental PVB19 infection occurs in about 30% (1990) to 50% of infected, previously sero-negative mothers (De Jong et al., 2012) (Gratacos et al., 1995) (Koch et al., 1998).

If fetal hydrops develops, the interval between the onset of infection and fetal diagnosis ranged from 2 to 6 weeks (Yaegashi et al., 1998). Adverse fetal outcome is increased when maternal infection occurs during the first 2 trimesters of pregnancy, with the highest risk being during weeks 9-16 of pregnancy (Makhseed et al., 1999), (Wattre et al., 1998), (Yaegashi et al., 1994), (Nyman et al., 2002); however it may also occur during the 3rd trimester (Skjoldebrand-Sparre et al., 2000). If infection occurs in the last two months the fetus is affected only rarely (Miller et al., 1998) (Yaegashi et al., 1998) (Enders et al., 2004).

Infectivity of the Virus

There are three main genotypes with genotype 1 responsible for the majority of human infections worldwide. However, there is no correlation between special sequences and specific disease symptoms (Gallinella et al., 2003). NS1, which is the main nonstructural protein in PVB19, induces cell death by apoptosis in erythroid-lineage cells by a pathway that involves caspase 3 (Moffatt et al., 1998). The virus has two capsid proteins VP1 and VP2. (Heegaard and Brown, 2002). The N-terminal amino acids of the VP1 is the receptor-binding domain for the PVB19 uptake (Leisi et al., 2016). PVB19 binds with the antigen Ku80 of the infected cell surface. Since human bone marrow erythroid cells with glycophorin A or CD36, are positive for cell-surface expression of Ku80, the virus has tropism for the red blood cells inhibiting the erythroid cell line differentiation (Munakata et al., 2005). Direct toxic cell injury or cytolytic effect of PVB19 as well as PVB19 - induced apoptosis is involved in the pathogenesis of fetal anemia. The PVB19 induces a cell cycle arrest at either Gap 1 (G1) or Gap 2 (G2) phase (Chisaka et al., 2003). The cytopathic effect of the PVB19 infection on the erythroid progenitor cells is manifested as giant pro-normoblasts seen by light microscopy. Cytotoxic ultrastructural changes that include pseudopod formation, marginated chromatin and virus particles in the nucleus can be observed by transmission Electron Microscopy (Young et al., 1984).

DIAGNOSIS OF MATERNAL AND FETAL INFECTION

A. *Immunological Assays:* Detection of the levels of IgM and IgG antibodies to PVB19 is the more common way of diagnosis of infection. IgM assays are reliable to detect a current or recent infection for about 2-3 months following the infection (Bruu and Nordbo, 1995). IgG rises about 10 -14 days following infection and apparently lasts for life (Modrow and Dorsch, 2002).
B. *Virus detection:* PVB19 can be detected by isolation of viral DNA by direct hybridization or by polymerase chain reaction (PCR), as PCR is 100-1000 times more sensitive than direct hybridization (Clewley, 1989). PCR analysis for PVB19 in maternal sera is diagnostic but less sensitive than amniotic fluid in which the DNA

concentrations were found to be 100 to 5,000 times higher. PCR in amniotic fluid was in direct correlation with the matching fetal serum concentrations among 3 fetuses evaluated between 16 to 27 weeks of gestation (Ishikawa et al., 2015), but had high sensitivity only during the viremic stage. The combination of serology and PCR in sera improves he diagnostic rate of viremia. For example, in a group of randomly selected pregnant women in Norway, 50 women (3.7% of the cohort) with seroconversion also had viral DNA in their sera; 20% of the children of the infected mothers had positive PCR in cord blood (Barlinn et al., 2017). Another group of 31 women (6.8% of the cohort) had seroconversion between 18 weeks of pregnancy and birth. Of them, 24.2% had the virus detected in cord blood (Barlinn et al., 2017). The advantage of the combined serologic and PCR evaluations in maternal sera was also shown in a group of 53 women infected during pregnancy. Among 37 with normal fetal ultrasonography, 78.3% had positive IgM while viral DNA was detected in 97.3%. Among the other 16 infected women whose fetuses developed signs of infection, IgM was detected only in 62.5%, while viral DNA was detected in 87.5%. Two of the fetuses developed hydrops fetalis, a third developed ascites and cardiac hypertrophy, one infant had hepatic calcifications, and one growth restriction (Zavattoni et al., 2016).

C. *Tests for discrimination of past from recent infection:* qPCR for determination of viral load may help in the staging of infection; however low viral loads may sometimes persist for life. A useful approach for such a differentiation is determination of maturing IgG avidity with assays using VP1u as the antigen. Low avidity correlates with recent infection and as the primary antibody response matures the antibody avidity increases (Soderlund et al., 1995). Another approach is the use of epitope type specificity enzyme immunoassay, which is based on the finding that antibodies to linear VP2 epitopes are mostly found during acute infections and early convalescence, while those to conformational epitopes persist through life (Maple et al., 2014).

D. *Diagnosis of fetal infection:* The prenatal diagnosis by IgM in fetal cord blood was found to have low sensitivity. IgM from fetal blood may give negative results despite fetal infection, since the fetus does not begin to make its own IgM until at least 22 weeks of gestation (Sifakis et al., 1998). PCR increases the accuracy of the diagnosis. However infection can be detected by PCR in the amniotic fluid or fetal serum mostly during the viremic stage. PVB19 infection can be diagnosed in the fetal tissues by identifying intranuclear inclusions or viral particles by electron microscopy (Crane et al., 2014).

Plasma cell-free RNA is a new non-invasive diagnostic tool that can reflect the dynamic changes of different tissues during pregnancy in both the mother and the fetus. It is derived from apoptotic bodies and exosomes, is highly degraded and usually has low quantity. However it can potentially be used as a more comprehensive screening test (Pan et al., 2017).

CONSEQUENCES OF FETAL INFECTION

Transplacental transmission of PVB19 may lead to fetal infection. Placental trophoblastic cells can express globoside which enables viral invasion. Immunohistochemical analysis revealed that poor outcome of PVB19-complicated pregnancies was associated with a higher rate of apoptosis among placental villous trophoblastic cells compared to those with good outcomes (Jordan and Butchko, 2002). Inflammation-mediated cellular immune responses within placentae from women whose pregnancies were complicated with PVB19 infection had an increase in CD3-positive T cells and IL2 levels. However, the presence of an inflammatory response was not associated with an increased risk of adverse pregnancy outcome (Jordan et al., 2001).

No clear association between PVB19 infection in pregnancy and early miscarriages was found in a literature review of studies published between 2009-2015 considering infections associated with miscarriages (Giakoumelou et al., 2016). A study from Norway, evaluating pregnancies complicated by PVB19 infection did not find increased rate of fetal death but found increased rate of low birth weight among still born infants (Sarfraz et al., 2009).

During the second trimester of pregnancy the liver is the main source of hematopoetic activity and the half- life of red blood cells is short, 50-75 days compared with later hematopoetic stages (Nyman et al., 2002). PVB19 induces apoptosis of the erythroid lineage cells of the fetal liver. Apoptosis induced by PVB19 was directly caused by the NS1 protein that was encoded by the viral genome (Yaegashi, 2000).

Cardiac failure resulting from severe anemia may be further aggravated by myocarditis. The P antigen expressed on fetal cardiac myocytes enables the PVB19 to directly infect myocardial cells (Rouger et al., 1987) (von Kaisenberg et al., 2001) (Morey et al., 1992) (Wang et al., 1999).

PVB19 infection may be associated with cases of nonhydropic intrauterine fetal death. Severe fetal damage can occur from the damage to different cell lines. Globoside, the cellular receptor necessary for B19 infectivity, is characteristic of the erythroid precursor cells. However, other non-erythroid cells can express this receptor and be infected by PVB19 including megakaryocytes, endothelial cells, cardiac myocytes and placental trophoblastic cells (Jordan and Butchko, 2002).

Fetal PVB19 infection can be complicated by thrombocytopenia. Severely thrombocytopenic fetuses were characterized by lower hemoglobin concentrations, lower reticulocyte count, lower gestational age at the time of diagnosis, increased fetal death rate and risk of prematurity. Fetal thrombocytopenia was more common during the second trimester but, in some cases, persisted into the third trimester. Intrauterine transfusion with RBC resulted in a further decrease in fetal platelet concentration (Melamed et al., 2015).

HYDROPS FETALIS DUE TO PVB19 INTRAUTERINE INFECTION

Hydrops Fetalis is the main fetal life threatening complication of PVB19 infection. The term Hydrops fetalis is referred to fluid accumulation in at least two out of the pericardial, pleural abdominal and cutaneous fetal compartments. Skin edema is defined as skin thickness >5 mm. Polyhydramnios and edematous placenta (defined as placental thickness ≥4 cm in the second trimester or ≥ 6cm in the third trimester of pregnancy) are common but not mandatory finding. The pathophysiology underlying hydrops fetalis is increased interstitial fluid production and hence its accumulation, or decreased lymphatic return (Yaegashi, 2000). Hydrops fetalis may have either an immune or non-immune etiology (Izetbegovic, 2013). During the last years, non-immune hydrops fetalis (NIHF) accounts for about 90% of the cases of hydrops fetalis with a prevalence of 1 in 1700-3000 pregnancies (Society for Maternal-Fetal Medicine et al., 2015). However due to early miscarriages before ultrasonography is performed, the real incidence may be higher.

Diagnosis of the etiology of NIHF includes fetal ultrasonography, echocardiography and invasive testing for karyotype and special DNA, and PCR testing for specific anomalies and infections. The main etiologies for NIHF are: cardiovascular: 17-35%; chromosomal: 7-16%; infectious: 5-7%; thoracic: 6%; twin to twin transfusion syndrome (TTTS): 3-10%; lymphatic dysplasia: 5-6%; skeletal dysplasia and specific syndromes 3-4% each: gastrointestinal: 0.5-4%; tumors including chorioangiomas: 2-3%; inborn errors of metabolism: 1-2%; miscellaneous: 3-15% and unknown 15-25% (Society for Maternal-Fetal Medicine et al., 2015).

In most published studies, the reported prevalence PVB19 infection in fetuses with hydrops fetalis is less than 10%. For example, Hartge et al. (Hartge et al., 2015) found that 9/220 cases (4.1%) of hydrops had PVB19 infection. Among the 9 PVB19 cases, hydrops fetalis was diagnosed in the first trimester in 2 and in the second trimester in 7. Of the 9 pregnancies, only one infant survived. In a retrospective review of 92 pregnancies with

NIHF managed in Osaka, Japan, between 2000 and 2012, six had PVB19 infection (7%). Four were diagnosed in the first and two in the second trimester (Ota et al., 2016).

The interval between maternal PVB19 infection and diagnosis of hydrops fetalis was described as being 1-20 weeks, (Enders et al., 2004; Miller et al., 1998; Nunoue et al., 2002; Yaegashi et al., 1998), and the median interval is about 3 weeks. Early pregnancy loss is rarely accompanied by hydrops fetalis (Wright, 1998). Nonimmune hydrops fetalis was the main complication in 0.9% (Anderson and Cohen, 1987) (Hall, 1990) to 23% (Koch et al., 1998) of pregnancies among proven maternal infections with PVB19. The maximal risk for hydrops fetalis (7.1%) has been observed in pregnant women infected during gestational week 13-20 (Enders et al., 2004). Fetal loss occurred in 1.6% (Guidozzi et al., 1994) to 24% (Levy and Read, 1990). Non hydropic fetal loss in late gestation complicated by PVB19 was rarely described (Norbeck et al., 2002; Tolfvenstam et al., 2001) and is controversial (Sebire, 2001).

TREATMENT OF HYDROPS FETALIS

A. Intrauterine Transfusion

The recommended management of fetuses with hydrops or anemia due to PVB19 infection is cordocentesis in order to assess fetal hemoglobin and reticulocyte count, and intrauterine transfusion when necessary (Crane et al., 2014). For near term pregnancies, corticosteroids to accelerate lung maturation, followed by premature delivery can be considered.

Intrauterine packed red blood cell transfusions for cases of hydrops fetalis improves the anemia and may lead to resolution of fetal heart failure and edema (Rodis et al., 1998). Sometimes, intra-uterine transfusion may be required already in the second trimester of pregnancy when fetuses are especially sensitive to acute hemodynamic changes and there are difficulties in fetal vascular access.

Indications for intra-uterine RBC infusion are ultrasonographic signs of hydrops fetalis and increased peak systolic velocity in the middle cerebral artery (MCA-PSV) as diagnosed by Doppler ultrasound. MCA-PSV >1.5 multiples of the median for age is an indication for transfusion with 30-50 cc/kg of packed red blood cells. Some cases may need recurrent transfusions. This need is estimated by repeated ultrasonography, echocardiographic and Doppler studies. Transfusion is mostly carried out through the umbilical vein (85%), but can also be performed by intra-peritoneal (9.7%) and intra-cardiac (5.3%) approaches. There is about 80% survival rate. Most fetal deaths occur either during the procedure or the following day (Hellmund et al., 2017). In a meta-analysis of 14 studies comprising 1,436 cases of fetal PVB19 infection, the survival rate of transfused fetuses was 82% compared with 55% without transfusion. Two to three transfusions were required before resolution of the fetal hydrops or anemia, if it occurred at 3 to 12 weeks after the diagnosis (von Kaisenberg and Jonat, 2001). Garabedian (Garabedian et al., 2015) described the outcome of 10 fetuses treated with intrauterine RBC transfusion for hydrops fetalis due to PVB19 infection. They were all born on time with no need for further treatment; none of the children had anemia at birth and no neurological complications at their discharge from the hospital. Although rare, spontaneous resolution of the hydrops fetalis was reported (Rodis et al., 1998).

B. Immunological Treatment: Administration of Immunoglobulins

In non-severe cases, anti-PVB19 antibodies can be of clinical benefit. For example, improvement in fetal anemia and resolution of the ascites and pericardial effusion was observed two weeks after maternal supplementation with high-dose intravenous gamma globulin at 25 weeks of gestation (Selbing et al., 1995). Injection of PVB19-IgG-rich immunoglobulin into the peritoneal cavity of a fetus with hydrops fetalis was followed by a decrease in the viral DNA and resolution of fetal anemia and hydrops (Matsuda et al., 2005).

Human IgG monoclonal antibodies with potent neutralizing activity specific for VP1 and VP2, neutralized 50% of infectious PVB19 in vitro. Such antibodies are suggested as immunotherapy of acutely infected pregnant women; however no clinical approved product is available (Gigler et al., 1999).

Injuries to Different Fetal Organs

Structural anomalies in the offspring of mothers with PVB19 infection in pregnancy are rare. However, some fetuses and newborns infected by PV B19 were described with specific damage to several organs, suggesting a possible weak teratogenic potential of the virus.

A. Brain Injuries

Congenital hydrocephalus (2 cases) (Katz et al., 1996), cerebellar hemorrhage (2 cases) (Glenn et al., 2007), polymicrogyria (3 cases) (Pistorius et al., 2008) (Schulert et al., 2011) (Courtier et al., 2012) perivascular calcifications in the brain (one case) (Isumi et al., 1999) were reported among cases with proved PVB19 infection. Although the brain findings may be a coincidental unrelated event, the findings of 3 cases with polymicrogyria, point to the possibility that in rare cases the virus may specifically affect the cerebral cortex, presumably due to hypoxia (Courtier et al., 2012). In all three infected fetuses, fetal anemia and hydrops were also observed. Hence, it might indeed be relevant to perform a fetal brain MRI examination in fetuses affected by PVB19 with severe anemia and hydrops.

B. Gastrointestinal Injuries

Hyper echogenic bowel (Yaron et al., 1999), meconium peritonitis (Zerbini et al., 1998) (Schild et al., 1998) (Zerbini et al., 1993) and fetal liver calcifications (Simchen et al., 2002) were reported among fetuses with congenital PVB19 infection. Some cases of congenital hypoplasia of the abdominal muscles in newborns following intrauterine PVB19 infection complicated by hydrops fetalis were also reported (Travan et al., 2016), (Mace et al., 2011). However such hypoplasia was previously associated with fetal ascites from various other causes.

C. Ocular Injuries

Congenital corneal opacification (Plachouras et al., 1999), ocular malformations, extensive inflammatory reactions (Van Elsacker-Niele et al., 1989) and aphakic eyes were described among embryos infected with PVB19 during early pregnancy (Hartwig et al., 1988).

D. Cardiac Injuries

Ebstein's anomaly (White et al., 1995), muscular ventricular septal defect (Rogers et al., 1993), fetal second-degree heart block and cardiomyopathy (Fishman et al., 2011) were reported. It seems that these incidental cases are not due to the PVB19 infection. Indeed, the virus may cross the placenta and infect the heart muscle but apparently does not cause anatomical cardiac anomalies.

E. Other Structural Defects

Bilateral cleft lip and palate, micrognathia and arthrogryposis (1 case) (Tiessen et al., 1994), micropenis with perineoscrotal hypospadias, bifid scrotum and secundum atrial septal defect (1 case) (Konstantinidou et al., 2007), Hypospadias (2 cases) (Hall, 1990) were reported among fetuses infected with PV B19.

F. Genetic Aberrations and Increased Susceptibility to Damage by PVB19

Calsen et al. found among 57 cases of spontaneous abortions, fetal or neonatal death that 9 had intrauterine PVB19 infection. Of these, three fetuses with hydrops fetalis and one with teratoma of the neck were also diagnosed with trisomies. They hypothesize that fetuses with trisomy, similar to children, are also more susceptible to infections (Carlsen et al., 2010).

A new paragraph as this is a summary of the entire issue of anomalies

In summary: Fetal abnormalities associated with PVB19 are rare, but if present, they may be severe. The possible teratogenicity of the PVB19, especially affecting the brain, needs further evaluation.

Neurodevelopmental Effects of Prenatal PVB19 Infection

As stated above, PVB19 may induce, although rarely, severe pathological changes in the fetal brain. These changes may obviously have severe neurodevelopmental sequelae. However the main question is whether PVB19 may affect the long-term neurodevelopment even in cases without any evident neuropathological brain injuries.

There is insufficient data assessing the neurodevelopmental outcome of children with prenatal PVB19 infections. Most studies describe the neurodevelopmental effect of infected children who had hydrops fetalis and therefore had intrauterine transfusion. Some studies describe the outcome of children with non-immune hydrops in general, including PVB19 infections, and lack comparative control groups. Hence, the number of children studied is too small to come to any definite conclusion.

Miller et al. (Miller et al., 1998) were among the first that assessed, by using questionnaires, the developmental outcome of 129 school age children born to mothers with PVB19 infection during pregnancy. Their development was reported to be normal. However, these children were not examined by the investigators.

Dembinski et al. (Dembinski et al., 2002) examined 20 surviving children out of 31 that had intrauterine transfusion due to non- immune hydrops fetalis (NIHF) and whose mothers had PVB19 infection during pregnancy. The children were examined at the ages of 1 to 9 years. Their average IQ was 101 (84-116). Two children (10%), however, had IQ below 85. There was no comparative control group. Similarly, De Jong et al. (De Jong et al., 2012) studied a group of 28 children, 1.5-13 years of age, with maternal PVB19 infection that had NIHF and intrauterine blood transfusion, using age appropriate psychometric tests. The average IQ score was 102, range 20-128. Three of the 28 infants (10.7%) had severe neurodevelopmental delay, one of them also had cerebral palsy. Nagel et al. (Nagel et al., 2007) studied the developmental outcome of 16 survivors of intrauterine transfusion due to PVB19, with 5 (31%) having delayed psychomotor development, two children with severe delay and three with moderate delay. We found no additional cases. Hence, of 64 children, all survivors of intrauterine transfusion, 10 (15.6%) had significant neurodevelopmental problems. It is indeed difficult to know whether this, rather poor developmental outcome, is related to the intrauterine infection and anemia or to the fetal hydrops and blood transfusion. Hence, it is important to assess the neurodevelopmental outcome of children who had intrauterine transfusion for reasons other than PVB19 infection.

Neurodevelopmental Data on Intrauterine Transfusion Not Related to PVB19 Infections

There are many studies reporting the neurodevelopmental outcome of children that received intrauterine transfusions because of anemia, due to hemolytic disease or other problems, excluding PVB19 infections. Generally, the outcome seems to be quite favorable (Lindenburg et al., 2013). The outcome also depends on the degree of fetal anemia and whether fetal hydrops developed or not. For example: Hudon et al. (Hudon et al., 1998) evaluated the development of 40 children who had severe fetal hemolytic diseases and survived intrauterine blood transfusion and found normal cognitive indexes at 9-18 months of age and at 36-62 months. Only two children (5%) had severe neurodevelopmental problems.

Lindenburg et al. (Lindenburg et al., 2012) carried out neurodevelopmental studies on 291 children at 2-17 years of age born after intrauterine transfusion because of hemolytic disease. They found that only 4.8% had significant neurodevelopmental problems (CP, deafness, severe delay). Although intrauterine transfusion for fetal anemia was not associated with significant neurodevelopmental problems, the cases with hydrops fetalis in this group had a high rate of neurodevelopmental problems with an odds ratio of 11.2 (95% CI 1.7-92.7).

Harper et al. (Harper et al., 2006) studied the development of 16 children with immune hydrops fetalis and intrauterine transfusion and found 2 (12.5%) with major neurologic sequelae. Ota et al., in a recent publication (Ota et al., 2016) examined at one year of age 51 surviving children from 92 pregnancies with NIHF and intrauterine blood transfusion in Osaka Medical Center, of which only 2 were infected by PVB19. Only 15 (44%) of the 33 hydropic fetuses had normal development. However, many of those with developmental delay also had different chromosomal abnormalities that do not enable any conclusion as to the effects of hydrops/intrauterine transfusion on development.

In summary: In spite of the significant limitations of these studies and especially the low numbers, hydrops fetalis due to PVB19 infection seems to affect the neurodevelopmental abilities in up to 15% of cases. However, as neurodevelopmental problems were also observed in children born after fetal hydrops and intrauterine blood transfusion not infected by PVB19, it is unknown whether it results from the infection, from the hydrops and severe anemia or from the blood transfusion. In spite of the fact that the exact pathogenesis is unknown, the rate of neurodevelopmental sequelae in PVB19 infected fetuses with hydrops seems to be high and warrants serious consideration and additional studies.

Recommended Guidelines for PVB19 Infection in Pregnancy

Guidelines for prevention, evaluation and management of women who were exposed to PVB19 during pregnancy were published by the Canadian Maternal Fetal Medicine Committee (SOGC), in December 2014 (Crane et al., 2014), and by the American College of Obstetricians and Gynecologists (ACOG) (American College of and Gynecologists, 2015) in June 2015.

Most recommendations are similar. Routine screening for PVB19 immunity in low-risk pregnancies is not indicated. Women should be screened for PVB19 infection immediately after exposure, to assess their basic serology. If negative, they should be followed up. Screening should also be done when ultrasonography reveals hydrops fetalis. Pregnant women who are exposed to, or who develop symptoms of fetal PVB19 infection including: placentomegaly, fetal ascites, cardiomegaly, hydrops fetalis and impaired growth, should be assessed by determining their PVB19 IgG and IgM status.

If PVB19 IgG is positive and IgM is negative, the woman is immune and should be reassured that she will not develop infection. Women who are IgM positive should be monitored for potential fetal infection regardless of IgG status. Women who are IgM and IgG negative and are susceptible to PVB19 infection should be followed within 4 weeks. In case of positive IgM, serial ultrasonographies with Doppler measurement of the middle cerebral artery peak systolic velocity (as a measure of fetal anemia) should be performed every 1 to 2 weeks, up to 12 weeks after infection. In the absence of ultrasound evidence of fetal sequelae by 8–12 weeks after exposure, PVB19 infection is unlikely. If hydrops fetalis is present or severe fetal anemia is suspected, fetal infection can be diagnosed using PCR in amniotic fluid. Fetal blood sampling by cordocentesis should be performed to determine the fetal hematocrit and platelets count and consider intrauterine transfusion if severe fetal anemia is present.

Recommendations differ for the precautions measures. The SOGC recommends that during endemic periods women should be advised to minimize exposure at work and at home and absence from work should be considered, while the ACOG claims that exclusion from the workplace is not recommended.

Vaccine

A specific vaccine is important in order to prevent aplastic crises in patients with underlying disorders and fetal complications in sero-negative women at child-bearing age. Two vaccines developed based on VP1 and VP2 capsid proteins were immunogenic in phase 1 trials. However, the immunized persons suffered from headache, fever, gastrointestinal distress and fatigue (Ballou et al., 2003) in the first one and skin manifestations in the second (Bernstein et al., 2011). A new vaccine based on a saccharomyces cerevisiae-derived PVB19 virus-like-particle includes a point mutation in VP1 that eliminated its phospholipase A2 activity, a potential cause of the adverse reactions observed in the clinical trials. The vaccine was found immunogenic in mice (Chandramouli et al., 2013), including a mouse model for sickle cell disease (Penkert et al., 2017) but was not evaluated in a clinical trial among humans.

In conclusions: Parvovirus B19 infection during pregnancy is quite common, especially during epidemics. Fortunately, the effects on pregnancy outcome are relatively rare, but can be quite serious and even fatal to the fetus. The more common complications are severe anemia, thrombocytopenia, increased mid-trimester abortions and hydrops fetalis that may be fatal if untreated. Treatment is by intrauterine blood transfusion which has its complications. Various congenital anomalies, including serious brain lesions may occur, although rarely. The extent of the neurodevelopmental sequelae is still not clear, but they seem to exist in 10-15% of offspring who suffered from hydrops fetalis and intrauterine transfusion. In spite of the extent of the problems, there is still no effective vaccine against parvovirus, and no adequate possibility for prevention.

REFERENCES

Adam, O., Makkawi, T., Reber, U., Kirberg, H. & Eis-Hubinger, A. M. (2015). The seroprevalence of parvovirus B19 infection in pregnant women in Sudan. *Epidemiol Infect*, *143*(2), 242-248.

American College of O, Gynecologists. (2015). Practice bulletin no. 151: Cytomegalovirus, parvovirus B19, varicella zoster, and toxoplasmosis in pregnancy. *Obstet Gynecol*, *125*(6), 1510-1525.

Anderson, L. J. (1987). Role of parvovirus B19 in human disease. *Pediatr Infect Dis J*, *6*(8), 711-718.

Anderson, M. J. & Cohen, B. J. (1987). Human parvovirus B19 infections in United Kingdom 1984-86. *Lancet*, *1*(8535), 738-739.

Ballou, W. R., Reed, J. L., Noble, W., Young, N. S. & Koenig, S. (2003). Safety and immunogenicity of a recombinant parvovirus B19 vaccine formulated with MF59C.1. *J Infect Dis*, *187*(4), 675-678.

Barlinn, R., Rollag, H., Trogstad, L., Vainio, K., Basset, C., Magnus, P. & Dudman, S. G. (2017). High incidence of maternal parvovirus B19 infection in a large unselected population-based pregnancy cohort in Norway. *J Clin Virol*, *94*, 57-62.

Barros De Freitas, R., Buarque De Gusmao, S. R., Durigon, E. L. & Linhares, A. C. (1999). Survey of Parvovirus B19 Infection in a Cohort of Pregnant Women in Belem, Brazil. *Braz J Infect Dis*, *3*(1), 6-14.

Baschat, A. A., Towbin, J., Bowles, N. E., Harman, C. R. & Weiner, C. P. (2003). Prevalence of viral DNA in amniotic fluid of low-risk pregnancies in the second trimester. *J Matern Fetal Neonatal Med*, *13*(6), 381-384.

Bernstein, D. I., El Sahly, H. M., Keitel, W. A., Wolff, M., Simone, G., Segawa, C., Wong, S., Shelly, D., Young, N. S. & Dempsey, W. (2011). Safety and immunogenicity of a candidate parvovirus B19 vaccine. *Vaccine*, *29*(43), 7357-7363.

Bonvicini, F., Puccetti, C., Salfi, N. C., Guerra, B., Gallinella, G., Rizzo, N. & Zerbini, M. (2011). Gestational and fetal outcomes in B19 maternal infection: a problem of diagnosis. *J Clin Microbiol*, *49*(10), 3514-3518.

Bruu, A. L. & Nordbo, S. A. (1995). Evaluation of five commercial tests for detection of immunoglobulin M antibodies to human parvovirus B19. *J Clin Microbiol*, *33*(5), 1363-1365.

Carlsen, K., Beck, B. L., Bagger, P. V., Christensen, L. S. & Donders, G. G. (2010). Pregnancy loss ascribable to parvovirus B19/erythrovirus is associated with a high prevalence of trisomy. *Gynecol Obstet Invest*, *70*(4), 328-334.

Chandramouli, S., Medina-Selby, A., Coit, D., Schaefer, M., Spencer, T., Brito, L. A., Zhang, P., Otten, G., Mandl, C. W., Mason, P. W., Dormitzer, P. R. & Settembre, E. C. (2013). Generation of a parvovirus B19 vaccine candidate. *Vaccine*, *31*(37), 3872-3878.

Chisaka, H., Morita, E., Yaegashi, N. & Sugamura, K. (2003). Parvovirus B19 and the pathogenesis of anaemia. *Rev Med Virol*, *13*(6), 347-359.

Clewley, J. P. (1989). Polymerase chain reaction assay of parvovirus B19 DNA in clinical specimens. *J Clin Microbiol*, *27*(12), 2647-2651.

Courtier, J., Schauer, G. M., Parer, J. T., Regenstein, A. C., Callen, P. W. & Glenn, O. A. (2012). Polymicrogyria in a fetus with human parvovirus B19 infection: a case with radiologic-pathologic correlation. *Ultrasound Obstet Gynecol*, *40*(5), 604-606.

Crane, J., Mundle, W., Boucoiran, I., Maternal Fetal Medicine, C., Gagnon, R., Bujold, E., Basso, M., Bos, H., Brown, R., Cooper, S., Gouin, K., McLeod, N. L., Menticoglou, S., Mundle, W., Pylypjuk, C., Roggensack, A. & Sanderson, F. (2014). Parvovirus B19 infection in pregnancy. *J Obstet Gynaecol Can*, *36*(12), 1107-1116.

De Jong, E. P., Lindenburg, I. T., van Klink, J. M., Oepkes, D., van Kamp, I. L., Walther, F. J. & Lopriore, E. (2012). Intrauterine transfusion for parvovirus B19 infection: long-term neurodevelopmental outcome. *Am J Obstet Gynecol*, *206*(3), *204* e201-205.

Dembinski, J., Haverkamp, F., Maara, H., Hansmann, M., Eis-Hubinger, A. M. & Bartmann, P. (2002). Neurodevelopmental outcome after intrauterine red cell transfusion for parvovirus B19-induced fetal hydrops. *BJOG*, *109*(11), 1232-1234.

Di Domenico, C., Moschese, V., Chini, L., Zirletta, E., Cancrini, C., Di, Paolo, A., Rossi, P. & Scalamandre, A. (2002). [Perinatal infections of B19 Parvoviruses]. *Ig Sanita Pubbl L*, *VIII*(3), 155-162.

Disease PHLSWPoF. (1990). Prospective study of human parvovirus (B19) infection in pregnancy. Public Health Laboratory Service Working Party on Fifth Disease. *BMJ*, 300(6733), 1166-1170.

Enders, M., Weidner, A., Zoellner, I., Searle, K. & Enders, G. (2004). Fetal morbidity and mortality after acute human parvovirus B19 infection in pregnancy: prospective evaluation of 1018 cases. *Prenat Diagn*, 24(7), 513-518.

Fauquet, C. M. & Mayo, M. A. (2001). The 7th ICTV report. *Arch Virol*, 146(1), 189-194.

Fishman, S. G., Pelaez, L. M., Baergen, R. N. & Carroll, S. J. (2011). Parvovirus-mediated fetal cardiomyopathy with atrioventricular nodal disease. *Pediatr Cardiol*, *32*(1), 84-86.

Friese, K., Beichert, M., Hof, H., Weikel, W., Falke, D., Sickinger, R. & Melchert, F. (1991). [Incidence of congenital infections]. *Geburtshilfe Frauenheilkd*, *51*(11), 890-896.

Gallinella, G., Venturoli, S., Manaresi, E., Musiani, M. & Zerbini, M. (2003). B19 virus genome diversity: epidemiological and clinical correlations. *J Clin Virol*, *28*(1), 1-13.

Garabedian, C., Rakza, T., Thomas, D., Wibaut, B., Vaast, P., Subtil, D. & Houfflin-Debarge, V. (2015). Neonatal outcome after fetal anemia managed by intrauterine transfusion. *Eur J Pediatr*, *174*(11), 1535-1539.

Giakoumelou, S., Wheelhouse, N., Cuschieri, K., Entrican, G., Howie, S. E. & Horne, A. W. (2016). The role of infection in miscarriage. *Hum Reprod Update*, *22*(1), 116-133.

Gigler, A., Dorsch, S., Hemauer, A., Williams, C., Kim, S., Young, N. S., Zolla-Pazner, S., Wolf, H., Gorny, M. K. & Modrow S. (1999). Generation of neutralizing human monoclonal antibodies against parvovirus B19 proteins. *J Virol*, *73*(3), 1974-1979.

Gilarranz, R., Chamizo, F., Hernandez-Febles, M., Valle, L. & Pena-Lopez, M. J. (2016). Parvovirus B19 congenital infection. *Infect Dis (Lond)*, *48*(7), 566-568.

Glenn, O. A., Bianco, K., Barkovich, A. J., Callen, P. W. & Parer, J. T. (2007). Fetal cerebellar hemorrhage in parvovirus-associated non-immune hydrops fetalis. *J Matern Fetal Neonatal Med*, *20*(10), 769-772.

Gratacos, E., Torres, P. J., Vidal, J., Antolin, E., Costa, J., Jimenez de Anta, M. T., Cararach, V., Alonso, P. L. & Fortuny, A. (1995). The incidence of human parvovirus B19 infection during pregnancy and its impact on perinatal outcome. *J Infect Dis*, *171*(5), 1360-1363.

Guidozzi, F., Ballot, D. & Rothberg, A. D. (1994). Human B19 parvovirus infection in an obstetric population. A prospective study determining fetal outcome. *J Reprod Med*, *39*(1), 36-38.

Hall, S. M. (1990). Prospective study of human parvovirus (B19) infection in pregnancy. Public Health Laboratory Service Working Party on Fifth Disease. *BMJ*, *300*(6733), 1166-1170.

Harper, D. C., Swingle, H. M., Weiner, C. P., Bonthius, D. J., Aylward, G. P. & Widness, J. A. (2006). Long-term neurodevelopmental outcome and brain volume after treatment for hydrops fetalis by in utero intravascular transfusion. *Am J Obstet Gynecol*, *195*(1), 192-200.

Hartge, DR., Weichert, J., Gembicki, M., Krapp M. (2015). Confirmation of etiology in fetal hydrops by sonographic evaluation of fluid allocation patterns. *Eur J Obstet Gynecol Reprod Biol*, *195*, 128-132.

Hartwig, N. G., Vermeij-Keers, C. & Versteeg, J. (1988). The anterior eye segment in virus induced primary congenital aphakia. *Acta Morphol Neerl Scand*, *26*(4), 283-292.

Heegaard, E. D. & Brown, K. E. (2002). Human parvovirus B19. *Clin Microbiol Rev*, *15*(3), 485-505.

Hellmund, A., Geipel, A., Berg, C., Bald, R. & Gembruch, U. (2017). Early Intrauterine Transfusion in Fetuses with Severe Anemia Caused by Parvovirus B19 Infection. *Fetal Diagn Ther*.

Hudon, L., Moise, K. J., Jr., Hegemier, S. E., Hill, R. M., Moise, A. A., Smith, E. O. & Carpenter, R. J. (1998). Long-term neurodevelopmental outcome after intrauterine transfusion for the treatment of fetal hemolytic disease. *Am J Obstet Gynecol*, *179*(4), 858-863.

Ishikawa, A., Yoto, Y., Asakura, H. & Tsutsumi, H. (2015). Quantitative analysis of human parvovirus B19 DNA in maternal and fetal serum, and amniotic fluid during an early stage of pregnancy. *J Med Virol*, *87*(4), 683-685.

Isumi, H., Nunoue, T., Nishida, A. & Takashima, S. (1999). Fetal brain infection with human parvovirus B19. *Pediatr Neurol*, *21*(3), 661-663.

Izetbegovic, S. (2013). Occurrence of ABO And RhD Incompatibility with Rh Negative Mothers. *Mater Sociomed*, *25*(4), 255-258.

Jensen, I. P., Thorsen, P., Jeune, B., Moller, B. R. & Vestergaard, B. F. (2000). An epidemic of parvovirus B19 in a population of 3,596 pregnant women: a study of sociodemographic and medical risk factors. *BJOG*, *107*(5), 637-643.

Jordan, J., Tiangco, B., Kiss, J. & Koch, W. (1998). Human parvovirus B19: prevalence of viral DNA in volunteer blood donors and clinical outcomes of transfusion recipients. *Vox Sang*, *75*(2), 97-102.

Jordan, J. A. & Butchko, A. R. (2002). Apoptotic activity in villous trophoblast cells during B19 infection correlates with clinical outcome: assessment by the caspase-related M30 Cytodeath antibody. *Placenta*, *23*(7), 547-553.

Jordan, J. A., Huff, D. & DeLoia, J. A. (2001). Placental cellular immune response in women infected with human parvovirus B19 during pregnancy. *Clin Diagn Lab Immunol*, *8*(2), 288-292.

Katz, V. L., McCoy, M. C., Kuller, J. A. & Hansen, W. F. (1996). An association between fetal parvovirus B19 infection and fetal anomalies: a report of two cases. *Am J Perinatol*, 13(1), 43-45.

Kerr, J. R., O'Neill, H. J., Coyle, P. V. & Thompson, W. (1994). An outbreak of parvovirus B19 infection; a study of clinical manifestations and the incidence of fetal loss. *Ir J Med Sci*, *163*(2), 65-67.

Koch, W. C. & Adler, S. P. (1989). Human parvovirus B19 infections in women of childbearing age and within families. *Pediatr Infect Dis J*, *8*(2), 83-87.

Koch, W. C., Harger, J. H., Barnstein, B. & Adler, S. P. (1998). Serologic and virologic evidence for frequent intrauterine transmission of human parvovirus B19 with a primary maternal infection during pregnancy. *Pediatr Infect Dis J*, *17*(6), 489-494.

Konstantinidou, A. E., Syridou, G., Spanakis, N., Tsakris, A., Agrogiannis, G. & Patsouris, E. (2007). Association of hypospadias and cardiac defect in a Parvovirus B19-infected stillborn: a causality relation? *J Infect*, *54*(1), e41-45.

Leisi, R., Di Tommaso, C., Kempf, C. & Ros, C. (2016). The Receptor-Binding Domain in the VP1u Region of Parvovirus B19. *Viruses*, *8*(3).

Levy, M. & Read, S. E. (1990). Erythema infectiosum and pregnancy-related complications. *Cmaj*, *143*(9), 849-858.

Lindenburg, I. T., Smits-Wintjens, V. E., van Klink, J. M., Verduin, E., van Kamp, I. L., Walther, F. J., Schonewille, H., Doxiadis., I. I., Kanhai, H. H., van Lith, J. M., van Zwet, E. W., Oepkes, D., Brand, A. & Lopriore, E., group Ls. (2012). Long-term neurodevelopmental outcome after intrauterine transfusion for hemolytic disease of the fetus/newborn: the LOTUS study. *Am J Obstet Gynecol*, *206*(2), 141 e141-148.

Lindenburg, I. T., van Klink, J. M., Smits-Wintjens, V. E., van Kamp, I. L., Oepkes, D. & Lopriore, E. (2013). Long-term neurodevelopmental and cardiovascular outcome after intrauterine transfusions for fetal anaemia: a review. *Prenat Diagn*, *33*(9), 815-822.

Mace, G., Audry, G., Cortey, A., Nguyen, A., Slaim, L., Castaigne, V., Garel, C. & Carbonne, B. (2011). Congenital hypoplasia of the abdominal wall muscles following fetal ascites due to parvovirus B19 infection. *Ultrasound Obstet Gynecol*, *37*(4), 497-498.

Makhseed, M., Pacsa, A., Ahmed, M. A. & Essa, S. S. (1999). Pattern of parvovirus B 19 infection during different trimesters of pregnancy in Kuwait. *Infect Dis Obstet Gynecol*, *7*(6), 287-292.

Maple, P. A., Hedman, L., Dhanilall, P., Kantola, K., Nurmi, V., Soderlund-Venermo, M., Brown, K. E. & Hedman, K. (2014). Identification of past and recent parvovirus B19 infection in immunocompetent individuals by quantitative PCR and enzyme immunoassays: a dual-laboratory study. *J Clin Microbiol*, *52*(3), 947-956.

Matsuda, H., Sakaguchi, K., Shibasaki, T., Takahashi, H., Kawakami, Y. & Furuya, K. (2005). Intrauterine therapy for parvovirus B19 infected symptomatic fetus using B19 IgG-rich high titer gammaglobulin. *J Perinat Med*, *33*(6), 561-563.

Melamed, N., Whittle, W., Kelly, E. N., Windrim, R., Seaward, P. G., Keunen, J., Keating, S. & Ryan, G. (2015). Fetal thrombocytopenia in pregnancies with fetal human parvovirus-B19 infection. *Am J Obstet Gynecol*, *212*(6), 793 e791-798.

Miller, E., Fairley, C. K., Cohen, B. J. & Seng, C. (1998). Immediate and long term outcome of human parvovirus B19 infection in pregnancy. *Br J Obstet Gynaecol*, *105*(2), 174-178.

Modrow, S. & Dorsch S. (2002). Antibody responses in parvovirus B19 infected patients. *Pathol Biol (Paris)*, *50*(5), 326-331.

Moffatt, S., Yaegashi, N., Tada, K., Tanaka, N. & Sugamura, K. (1998). Human parvovirus B19 nonstructural (NS1) protein induces apoptosis in erythroid lineage cells. *J Virol*, *72*(4), 3018-3028.

Morey, A. L., Keeling, J. W., Porter, H. J. & Fleming, K. A. (1992). Clinical and histopathological features of parvovirus B19 infection in the human fetus. *Br J Obstet Gynaecol*, *99*(7), 566-574.

Munakata, Y., Saito-Ito, T., Kumura-Ishii, K., Huang, J., Kodera, T., Ishii, T., Hirabayashi, Y., Koyanagi, Y. & Sasaki, T. (2005). Ku80 autoantigen as a cellular coreceptor for human parvovirus B19 infection. *Blood*, *106*(10), 3449-3456.

Nagel, H. T., de Haan, T. R., Vandenbussche, F. P., Oepkes, D. & Walther, F. J. (2007). Long-term outcome after fetal transfusion for hydrops associated with parvovirus B19 infection. *Obstet Gynecol*, *109*(1), 42-47.

Norbeck, O., Papadogiannakis, N., Petersson, K., Hirbod, T., Broliden, K. & Tolfvenstam, T. (2002). Revised clinical presentation of parvovirus B19-associated intrauterine fetal death. *Clin Infect Dis*, *35*(9), 1032-1038.

Nunoue, T., Kusuhara, K. & Hara, T. (2002). Human fetal infection with parvovirus B19: maternal infection time in gestation, viral persistence and fetal prognosis. *Pediatr Infect Dis J*, *21*(12), 1133-1136.

Nyman, M., Tolfvenstam, T., Petersson, K., Krassny, C., Skjoldebrand-Sparre, L. & Broliden, K. (2002). Detection of human parvovirus B19 infection in first-trimester fetal loss. *Obstet Gynecol*, *99*(5 Pt 1), 795-798.

Ota, S., Sahara, J., Mabuchi, A., Yamamoto, R., Ishii, K. & Mitsuda, N. (2016). Perinatal and one-year outcomes of non-immune hydrops fetalis by etiology and age at diagnosis. *J Obstet Gynaecol Res*, *42*(4), 385-391.

Pan, W., Ngo, T. T. M., Camunas-Soler, J., Song, C. X., Kowarsky, M., Blumenfeld, Y. J., Wong, R. J., Shaw, G. M., Stevenson, D. K. & Quake, S. R. (2017). Simultaneously Monitoring Immune Response and Microbial Infections during Pregnancy through Plasma cfRNA Sequencing. *Clin Chem*, *63*(11), 1695-1704.

Penkert, R. R., Young, N. S., Surman, S. L., Sealy, R. E., Rosch, J., Dormitzer, P. R., Settembre, E. C., Chandramouli, S., Wong, S., Hankins, J. S. & Hurwitz, J. L. (2017). Saccharomyces cerevisiae-derived virus-like particle parvovirus B19 vaccine elicits binding and neutralizing antibodies in a mouse model for sickle cell disease. *Vaccine*, *35*(29), 3615-3620.

Pistorius, L. R., Smal, J., de Haan, T. R., Page-Christiaens, G. C., Verboon-Maciolek, M., Oepkes, D. & de Vries, L. S. (2008). Disturbance of cerebral neuronal migration following congenital parvovirus B19 infection. *Fetal Diagn Ther*, *24*(4), 491-494.

Plachouras, N., Stefanidis, K., Andronikou, S. & Lolis, D. (1999). Severe nonimmune hydrops fetalis and congenital corneal opacification secondary to human parvovirus B19 infection. A case report. *J Reprod Med*, 44(4), 377-380.

Rodis, J. F., Borgida, A. F., Wilson, M., Egan, J. F., Leo, M. V., Odibo, A. O. & Campbell, W. A. (1998). Management of parvovirus infection in pregnancy and outcomes of hydrops: a survey of members of the Society of Perinatal Obstetricians. *Am J Obstet Gynecol*, *179*(4), 985-988.

Rogers, B. B., Mark, Y. & Oyer, C. E. (1993). Diagnosis and incidence of fetal parvovirus infection in an autopsy series: I. Histology. *Pediatr Pathol*, *13*(3), 371-379.

Rouger, P., Gane, P. & Salmon, C. (1987). Tissue distribution of H, Lewis and P antigens as shown by a panel of 18 monoclonal antibodies. *Rev Fr Transfus Immunohematol*, *30*(5), 699-708.

Sarfraz, A. A., Samuelsen, S. O., Bruu, A. L., Jenum, P. A. & Eskild, A. (2009). Maternal human parvovirus B19 infection and the risk of fetal death and low birthweight: a case-control study within 35 940 pregnant women. *BJOG*, *116*(11), 1492-1498.

Schild, R. L., Plath, H., Thomas, P., Schulte-Wissermann, H., Eis-Hubinger, A. M. & Hansmann, M. (1998). Fetal parvovirus B19 infection and meconium peritonitis. *Fetal Diagn Ther*, *13*(1), 15-18.

Schulert, G. S., Walsh, W. F. & Weitkamp, J. H. (2011). Polymicrogyria and congenital parvovirus b19 infection. *AJP Rep*, *1*(2), 105-110.

Sebire, N. J. (2001). Human parvovirus B19 and fetal death. *Lancet*, *358*(9288), 1180.

Selbing, A., Josefsson, A., Dahle, L. O. & Lindgren, R. (1995). Parvovirus B19 infection during pregnancy treated with high-dose intravenous gammaglobulin. *Lancet*, *345*(8950), 660-661.

Sifakis, S., Ergazaki, M., Sourvinos, G., Koffa, M., Koumantakis, E. & Spandidos, D. A. (1998). Evaluation of Parvo B19, CMV and HPV viruses in human aborted material using the polymerase chain reaction technique. *Eur J Obstet Gynecol Reprod Biol*, *76*(2), 169-173.

Simchen, M. J., Toi, A., Bona, M., Alkazaleh, F., Ryan, G. & Chitayat, D. (2002). Fetal hepatic calcifications: prenatal diagnosis and outcome. *Am J Obstet Gynecol*, *187*(6), 1617-1622.

Skjoldebrand-Sparre, L., Tolfvenstam, T., Papadogiannakis, N., Wahren, B., Broliden, K. & Nyman, M. (2000). Parvovirus B19 infection: association with third-trimester intrauterine fetal death. *Bjog*, *107*(4), 476-480.

Society for Maternal-Fetal, M., Norton, M. E., Chauhan, S. P. & Dashe, J. S. (2015). Society for maternal-fetal medicine (SMFM) clinical guideline #7: nonimmune hydrops fetalis. *Am J Obstet Gynecol*, *212*(2), 127-139.

Soderlund, M., Brown, C. S., Cohen, B. J. & Hedman K. (1995). Accurate serodiagnosis of B19 parvovirus infections by measurement of IgG avidity. *J Infect Dis*, *171*(3), 710-713.

Tiessen, R. G., van Elsacker-Niele, A. M., Vermeij-Keers, C., Oepkes, D., van Roosmalen, J. & Gorsira, M. C. (1994). A fetus with a parvovirus B19 infection and congenital anomalies. *Prenat Diagn*, *14*(3), 173-176.

Tolfvenstam, T., Papadogiannakis, N., Norbeck, O., Petersson, K. & Broliden, K. (2001). Frequency of human parvovirus B19 infection in intrauterine fetal death. *Lancet*, *357*(9267), 1494-1497.

Travan, L., Naviglio, S., Cont, G., Brovedani, P., Davanzo, R. & Demarini, S. (2016). Isolated hypoplasia of abdominal wall muscles associated with fetal ascites. *Congenit Anom* (Kyoto).

Valeur-Jensen, A. K., Pedersen, C. B., Westergaard, T., Jensen, I. P., Lebech, M., Andersen, P. K., Aaby, P., Pedersen, B. N. & Melbye, M. (1999). Risk factors for parvovirus B19 infection in pregnancy. *JAMA*, *281*(12), 1099-1105.

Van Elsacker-Niele, A. M., Salimans, M. M., Weiland, H. T., Vermey-Keers, C., Anderson, M. J. & Versteeg, J. (1989). Fetal pathology in human parvovirus B19 infection. *Br J Obstet Gynaecol*, *96*(7), 768-775.

von Kaisenberg, C. S., Bender, G., Scheewe, J., Hirt, S. W., Lange, M., Stieh, J., Kramer, H. H. & Jonat, W. (2001). A case of fetal parvovirus B19 myocarditis, terminal cardiac heart failure, and perinatal heart transplantation. *Fetal Diagn Ther*, *16*(6), 427-432.

von Kaisenberg, C. S. & Jonat, W. (2001). Fetal parvovirus B19 infection. *Ultrasound Obstet Gynecol*, *18*(3), 280-288.

Wang, X., Zhang, G., Han, M., Chao, Q. & Xu, D. (1999). Investigation of parvovirus B19 in cardiac tissue from patients with congenital heart disease. *Chin Med J (Engl)*, *112*(11), 995-997.

Wattre, P., Dewilde, A., Subtil, D., Andreoletti, L. & Thirion, V. (1998). A clinical and epidemiological study of human parvovirus B19 infection in fetal hydrops using PCR Southern blot hybridization and chemiluminescence detection. *J Med Virol*, *54*(2), 140-144.

White, F. V., Jordan, J., Dickman, P. S. & Knisely, A. S. (1995). Fetal parvovirus B19 infection and liver disease of antenatal onset in an infant with Ebstein's anomaly. *Pediatr Pathol Lab Med*, *15*(1), 121-129.

Woernle, C. H., Anderson, L. J., Tattersall, P. & Davison, J. M. (1987). Human parvovirus B19 infection during pregnancy. *J Infect Dis*, *156*(1), 17-20.

Wright, C. (1998). Detection of parvovirus B19 in macerated fetal tissue using in situ hybridization. *J Clin Pathol*, *51*(3), 262.

Yaegashi, N. (2000). Pathogenesis of nonimmune hydrops fetalis caused by intrauterine B19 infection. *Tohoku J Exp Med*, *190*(2), 65-82.

Yaegashi, N., Niinuma, T., Chisaka, H., Watanabe, T., Uehara, S., Okamura, K., Moffatt, S., Sugamura, K. & Yajima, A. (1998). The incidence of, and factors leading to, parvovirus B19-related hydrops fetalis following maternal infection; report of 10 cases and meta-analysis. *J Infect*, *37*(1), 28-35.

Yaegashi, N., Okamura, K., Yajima, A., Murai, C. & Sugamura, K. (1994). The frequency of human parvovirus B19 infection in nonimmune hydrops fetalis. *J Perinat Med*, *22*(2), 159-163.

Yaron, Y., Hassan, S., Geva, E., Kupferminc, M. J., Yavetz, H. & Evans, M. I. (1999). Evaluation of fetal echogenic bowel in the second trimester. *Fetal Diagn Ther*, *14*(3), 176-180.

Young, N., Harrison, M., Moore, J., Mortimer, P. & Humphries, R. K. (1984). Direct demonstration of the human parvovirus in erythroid progenitor cells infected in vitro. *J Clin Invest*, *74*(6), 2024-2032.

Zavattoni, M., Paolucci, S., Sarasini, A., Tassis, B., Rustico, M., Quarenghi, A., Piralla, A. & Baldanti, F. (2016). Diagnostic and prognostic value of molecular and serological investigation of human parvovirus B19 infection during pregnancy. *New Microbiol*, *39*(3), 181-185.

Zerbini, M., Gentilomi, G. A., Gallinella, G., Morandi, R., Calvi, S., Guerra, B. & Musiani, M. (1998). Intra-uterine parvovirus B19 infection and meconium peritonitis. *Prenat Diagn*, *18*(6), 599-606.

Zerbini, M., Musiani, M., Gentilomi, G., Venturoli, S., Gallinella, G., Gibellini, D., Morandi, R., Guerra, B., Bovicelli, L. & La Placa, M.

(1993). Symptomatic parvovirus B19 infection of one fetus in a twin pregnancy. *Clin Infect Dis*, *17*(2), 262-263.

BIOGRAPHICAL SKETCH

Zivanit Ergaz

Affiliation: Hadassah Hebrew University Medical Center Jerusalem, Israel

Education:

1976 – 1981 Doctor of Medicine, The Hebrew University and Hadassah School of Medicine. Jerusalem, Israel

1982 – 1983 Rotating Internship, Ein Kerem and Mount Scopus, Hadassah University Hospitals, Jerusalem, Israel

1985 – 1989 Pediatric Residency, Hadassah University Hospital, mount Scopus, Jerusalem, Israel

1990 – 1992 Fellowship in Neonatal – Perinatal Medicine, Hadassah University Hospital, Mount Scopus, Jerusalem, Israe

Research and Professional Experience: Neonatology, Neonatal sepsis, teratology, oxidative stress

Professional Appointments:

Senior lecturer in pediatrics, Hadassah Hebrew University Medical Center

Head of neonatal unit, Hadassah Mt. Scopus, Hebrew University Medical Center

Publications from the Last 3 Years:

[1] Ergaz Zivanit, Guillemin Claire, Neeman-azulay Meytal, Weinstein-Fudim Liza, Stodgell J.Christopher, Miller K. Richard, Ornoy Asher (2014) Placental oxidative stress and decreased global DNA

methylation are corrected by copper in the Cohen Diabetic Rat, *Toxicology Applied Pharmacology* May 1;276(3):220-30

[2] Ergaz Z, Bar-Oz B, Vainer GW, Abu-Leil S, Simanovsky N, Diav-Citrin O. Congenital fulminant Caposiform hemangioendothelioma of the leg.(2014) *Reprod Toxicol* Dec; 50: 1-3.

[3] Petropoulos S, Guillemin C, Ergaz Z, Dimov S, Suderman M, Weinstein-Fudim L, Ornoy A, Szyf M (2015). Gestational Diabetes Alters Offspring DNA Methylation Profiles in Human and Rat: Identification of Key Pathways involved in Endocrine System Disorders, Insulin Signaling, Diabetes Signaling and IL-K Signaling. *Endocrinology* Jun; 156(6): 2222-38

[4] Zivanit Ergaz [PI] Shmuel Benenson, Noa Ofek-Shlomai, Sinan Abu-Leil, Benjamin Bar-Oz MD (2015) Prediction of late onset sepsis in very low birth weight infants by a software application- are we there yet? Harefuah, Jan 2016, special issue in *Neonatology*.

[5] Uri Dior, Ronit Margalit-Calderon, Smadar Eventov-Friedman, Zivanit Ergaz, Shay Porat, Moran Gil, Liron Kogan, Smadar Eventov-Friedman (2015). Very High Intrapartum Fever In Term Pregnancies and Adverse Obstetric and Neonatal Outcomes. *Neonatology* 2016; 109(1):62-8. doi: 10.1159/000440938

[6] Zivanit Ergaz, Meytal Neeman-azulay, Liza Weinstein-Fudim, Sarah Weksler-Zangen, Dana Shoshani-Dror, Moshe Szyf, Asher Ornoy (2015). Diabetes in the Cohen rat intensifies the fetal pancreatic damage induced by the diabetogenic high sucrose low copper diet. *Birth defects research B*. 2016 Jan 7. doi:10.1002/bdrb.21169.

[7] Ergaz Z, Benenson S, Ofek-Shlomai N, Abu-Leil S, Bar-Oz B. Prediction of late onset sepsis in very low birth weight infants by a software application-are we there yet?, *Harefuah*. 2016 Jan; 155(1):15-9, 68. Hebrew

[8] Ornoy A, Weinstein-Fudim L, Ergaz Z: Prenatal factors associated with autism spectrum disorder (ASD) (2015) *Reprod Toxicol*. 2015 Aug 15; 56: 155-69. doi: 10.1016/j.reprotox.2015.05.007. Epub 2015 May 27.

[9] Ergaz-Shaltiel Zivanit: Neonatal pulmonology (2016). *Int J Child Health Hum Dev*. (2016)

[10] Zivanit Ergaz, Liza Weinstein-Fudim, Asher Ornoy Genetic and non-genetic animal models for autism spectrum disorders (ASD).) *Reprod Toxicol*. 2016 Sep; 64: 116-40. doi: 10.1016/j.reprotox.2016.04.024. Epub 2016 Apr 30

[11] Asher Ornoy, Liza Weinstein-Fudim, Zivanit Ergaz: Genetic Syndromes, Maternal Diseases and Antenatal Factors Associated with Autism Spectrum Disorders (ASD). Front *Neurosci*. 2016 Jul 6;10:316. doi: 10.3389/fnins.2016.00316. eCollection 2016

[12] Asher Ornoy, Zivanit Ergaz, Parvovirus B19 infection during pregnancy and risks to the fetus. *Birth Defects Res*. 2017 Mar 15;109(5):311-323. doi: 10.1002/bdra.23588. Review

[13] Ornoy A, Weinstein-Fudim L, Ergaz Zivanit., Antidepressants, Antipsychotics, and Mood Stabilizers in Pregnancy: What Do We Know and How Should We Treat Pregnant Women with Depression, *Birth Defects Res*. 2017 Jul 17; 109(12):933-956. doi: 10.1002/bdr2.1079. Review

[14] Ergaz-Shaltiel Zivanit, Engel O, Erlichman I, Naveh Y, Schimmel MS, Tenenbaum A, Neonatal characteristics and perinatal complications in neonates with Down syndrome, *Am J Med Genet A*. 2017 May; 173(5): 1279-1286. doi: 10.1002/ajmg.a.38165. Epub 2017 Apr 6

[15] Christoph Bu¨ hrer, O¨ mer Erdeve, Anton van Kaam, Angelika, Berger, Evelyn Lechner, Benjamin Bar-Oz, Karel Allegaert, Tom Stiris, Istemi Han C¸ elik, Janet Berrington, on behalf of the REDEXAM study group, Sinan Abu-Leil, Benjamin, Bausenhardt, Christoph Czernik, Ug˘ ur Dilmen, Nicholas Embleton, Zivanit Ergaz-Shaltiel, Lara Garabedian, Iren Lok, Tone Nordvik, Wes Onland, Øivind Ringen, Thomas, Skeath, Oliver Wagner, N-terminal B-type natriuretic peptide urinary concentrations and retinopathy of prematurity, *Pediatr Res*. 2017 Jul 24. doi: 10.1038/pr.2017.179.

Asher Ornoy, MD

Affiliation: Laboratory of Teratology Department of Medical Neurobiology, Israel Canada Institute of Medical Research, Hebrew University Hadassah Medical School, Jerusalem, Israel

Education: MD from the Hebrew University Hadassah Medical School Jerusalem

Training in Pediatrics at Hadassah University hospital, Jerusalem

Training in Teratology in the US in Cincinnati Children's hospital and in Jefferson Medical School Philadelphia

Training in Pediatric Neurology and Child Development, Cincinnati Children's Hospital and Jerusalem

Business Address: Department of Medical Neurobiology, Hebrew University Hadassah Medical School, Hadassah Ein Kerem Jerusalem Israel.

Research Experience: research in the areas of: clinical teratology, child development, child rehabilitation, Embryology, Animal models of human diseases (diabetes, Autism). Over 320 publications in peer reviewed scientific journals, 5 books and monographs, over 60 chapters in books and proceedings related to these topics.

Currently: Professor (Emeritus) of Embryology, Teratology and Medical Neurobiology at the Hebrew University, Jerusalem.

Professional Appointments: 1988-Currently: head, Laboratory of Teratology, Hebrew University Hadassah Medical School.

1996-2013 Founder and head, Department of Child Development and Rehabilitation, Israeli Ministry of Health.

2013-2014: Founder and head, Division of Rehabilitation, Israeli Ministry of Health

Head or member of many National and International committees related to child development and rehabilitation or to Clinical Teratology.

Honors: *1968*: prize for excellent MD thesis

1974/75: Fulbright Hay Fellowship in Clinical Teratology, Cincinnati USA

1993: European Teratology Society prize for best scientific presentation

2008: Special recognition by the Minister of Health for extraordinary contribution to Medicine in Israel in the area of Child Development and Rehabilitation.

2009: Special recognition by the School of occupational Therapy, Hebrew University and Hadassah for contribution to the School.

2012 Special recognition_by the Israeli Society for child development and rehabilitation for extraordinary and lifetime contribution to Child Development in Israel.

Publications from the Last 3 Years: 2015-2017

[1] Petropoulos S, Guillemin C, Ergaz Z, Dimov S, Suderman M, Weinstein-Fudim L, Ornoy A, Szyf M. Gestational Diabetes Alters Offspring DNA Methylation Profiles in Human and Rat: Identification of Key Genes involved in Endocrine System Disorders, Insulin Signaling, Diabetes Signaling and IL-K Signaling Pathways. *Endocrinology*, 156(6):2222-2238, 2015.

[2] Dvela-Levitt M, Cohen-Ben Ami H, Rosen H, Ornoy A, Hochner-Celnikier D, Granat M, Lichtstein D. Reduction in Maternal Circulating Ouabain Impairs Offspring Growth and Kidney Development. *J. Am. Soc. Nephrol.* 26(5):1103-1114, 2015.

[3] Ornoy A, Reece AE, Pavlinkova G, Kappen C, Miller RK. Effect of maternal diabetes on the embryo, fetus and children: congenital anomalies, genetic and epigenetic changes and developmental outcomes. *Birth Defects Res. Part C*, 105(1) 53-72, 2015.

[4] Aharon Hagai, Orna Diav-Citrin, Svetlana Shechtman, Asher Ornoy. Pregnancy outcome after in-utero exposure to local anesthetics as part of dental treatment: A prospective controlled cohort study. *Journal of the American Dental Association (J.A.D.A),* 146(8): 572-580, 2015.

[5] Ornoy A, Weinstein-Fudim L, Ergaz Z. Prenatal factors associated with autism spectrum disorder (ASD). *Reprod. Toxicol.* 56: 155-169, 2015.

[6] Hagai A, Diav-Citrin O, Shechtman S, Ornoy A. Authors response: *J Am Dent Assoc.* 146(12):868, 2015.

[7] Hagai A, Diav-Citrin O, Shechtman S, Ornoy A. Authors response. *J Am Dent Assoc*. 146(12):869-870, 2015.

[8] Diav-Citrin O, Shechtman S, Arnon J, Wajnberg R, Borisch C, Richardson JL, Bozzo P, Nulman I, Ornoy A. Methylphenidate in pregnancy: A multicenter, prospective, comparative, observational study. *The Journal of Clinical Psychiatry*, 77(9):1176-1181, 2016.

[9] Ergaz Z, Neeman-Azulay M, Weinstein-Fudim L, Weksler-Zangen **S,** Shoshani-Dror D, Szyf M, Ornoy A. Diabetes in the Cohen rat intensifies the fetal pancreatic damage induced by the diabetogenic high sucrose low copper diet. *Birth Defects Res. Part B, Developmental and Reproductive Toxicology*. 107(1):21-31 2016.

[10] Ornoy A, Finkel –Pekarsky V, Peles E, Adelson M, Schreiber S, Ebstein RP. ADHD risk alleles associated with opiate addiction: study of addicted parents and their children. *Ped. Res*. 80(2): 228-236, 2016.

[11] Ergaz Z, Fudim –Weinstein L, Ornoy A. Genetic and non-genetic animal models for Autism Spectrum Disorders (ASD) *Reproductive Toxicology*, 64: 116-140, 2016.

[12] Ornoy A, Ovadia M, Rivkin D, Milshtein E, Barlev L. Prevalence of ADHD among 7-9 years old children in Israel. A comparison between the Jewish and Arab populations. *Isr. J. Psychiatry*. 53(2): 3-8, 2016.

[13] Ornoy A, Weinstein– Fudim L, Ergaz Z. Genetic syndromes, maternal diseases and antenatal factors associated with Autism Spectrum Disorders (ASD). *Frontiers in Neurosci*. July 2016, 10:316. doi: 10.3389/fnins.2016.00316.

[14] Ornoy A, Ergaz Z. Parvovirus B19 infection during pregnancy and risks to the fetus. *Birth Defects Res. Part A: Clinical and Molecular Teratology*; 109(5):311-323 2017.

[15] Ornoy A. Neurobehavioral risks of SSRIs in pregnancy: comparing human and animal data. *Reprod. Toxicol*. 72:191-200, 2017**.**

[16] Ornoy A, Weinstein –Fudim L, Ergaz Z. Antidepressants, antipsychotics and mood stabilizers in pregnancy: what do we know and how should we treat pregnant women with depression. *Birth Defects Research Part C*. 109(12):933-956, 2017.

[17] Ornoy A, Koren G. Selective Serotonin Reuptake Inhibitors during pregnancy: do we have now more definite answers related to prenatal exposure. *Birth Defects Research Part C.* 109(12):898-908, 2017.

[18] Howdeshell, K, Ornoy, A. Depression and its treatment during pregnancy: Overview and Highlights *Birth Defects Research Part C.* 109(12):877-878, 2017.

[19] Diav-Citrin O, Shechtman S, Zvi N, Victoriya Finkel-Pekarsky V, Ornoy A. Is it safe to use lamotrigine during pregnancy? A prospective comparative observational study. *Birth Defects Res. Part A*, 109:1196–1203, 2017.

[20] Tal Saban M, Ornoy A, Parush S. Success in Adults with Probable DCD Using Structural Equation Modeling (SEM). *Am. J. Occup. Therapy*, 2017, in press.

[21] Ornoy A, Rivkin D, Barlev L. Diagnosis and treatment of children with ADHD: accessibility and availability of services and a comparison between treated and non-treated children in functioning and consumption of health services. *Harefuah*, 2017, in press

[22] Ornoy A. Pharmacological treatment of Attention Deficit Hyperactivity Disorder during pregnancy and lactation. *Pharmaceutical Research*, 2018, in press.

In: Advances in Health and Disease. Volume 4 ISBN: 978-1-53613-345-5
Editor: Lowell T. Duncan

Chapter 3

THE ROLE OF THERAPEUTIC DRUG MONITORING FOR TNF INHIBITORS IN IBD: SELECTED CASES OR EVERYDAY PRACTICE?

Lorant Gonczi*[1], *MD, Zsuzsanna Vegh*[1], *MD, Zsuzsanna Kurti*[1], *MD, Akos Ilias, MD*[1] *and Peter L. Lakatos*[1,2,*], *MD, DSc

[1]Semmelweis University, First Department of Internal Medicine, Budapest, Hungary

[2]McGill University, Division of Gastroenterology, Montreal, Canada

---

[*] Corresponding Author: Peter L. Lakatos, MD, DSc, FEBG, AGAF.

Director of IBD Centre, Associate Professor, McGill University, MUHC, Montreal General Hospital, 1650 Ave. Cedar, D16.173.1,Montreal, QC, H3G 1A4; Tel: +1-514-9341934 x ext 45567; Fax: +1-514-934-4452; Tel: +1-514-4317994; e-mail: Peter.Lakatos@muhc.mcgill.ca.

Associate Professor, Head of Gastroenterology/Hepatology Unit and Endoscopy, Semmelweis University, Koranyi S 2A, Budapest, H-1083, Hungary. Tel: +36-1-4591500/51500, 51520; Fax: +36-1-313-0250; e-mail: lakatos.peter_laszlo@med.semmelweis-univ.hu; e-mail: kislakpet99@gmail.com.

Abstract

Over the past 15 years, tumor necrosis factor (TNF) antagonists have revolutionized therapy for inflammatory bowel disease (IBD). Yet, a significant proportion of patients does not respond or lose effect to anti-TNF therapy over time. A 'tailored' treatment approach for anti-TNF treatment optimization has been suggested. Patient characterization is important prior and during therapy, multiple factors should be evaluated including clinical and disease characteristics, genetic factors and therapeutic drug monitoring (TDM) measuring anti-TNF drug levels and anti-drug antibodies (ADA). TDM can aid therapeutic decisions during primary and secondary treatment failure to anti-TNF treatment or proactive optimization of long-term disease management. TDM is routinely applied in the evaluation of secondary loss of response. The TDM-based strategy has several advantages over an empiric approach as it avoids unnecessary dose intensification, allows targeted switching between anti-TNF agents or out of class, and optimizes health care resources. Proactive TDM-based strategy to prevent anti-TNF treatment failure has also been suggested/investigated. However, routine monitoring of trough anti-TNF drug concentrations and targeted dose optimization had no additional benefit with regards to 1-year clinical outcome over strict clinical/biochemical based patient monitoring as observed in the TAXIT and TAILORIX trials. Of note, the TDM-based strategy of the TAXIT trial was associated with significantly fewer disease flares. Emerging data are published from real life cohorts, including, e.g., Belgium, The Netherlands, U.S., Denmark, France and Hungary supporting the case for TDM assessment at loss of response leading to earlier optimization of medical therapy and cost reduction, while further evidence is needed on the additional value of proactive TDM. This book chapter summarizes the evidence on the use of TDM in anti-TNF therapy to guide interventions at therapeutic failure, while present data do not support the routine use of proactive TDM in everyday clinical practice.

Introduction

Anti-tumor necrosis factor (TNF) therapies are proved to be effective and revolutionized the treatment of inflammatory bowel diseases (IBD). Goals of therapy and management have also changed in the past decade including both Crohn's disease (CD) and ulcerative colitis (UC). Treatment failure in patients treated with biologicals may occur as primary non-response (PNR) or secondary loss of response (LOR) which requires dose-intensification, switch or discontinuation of the therapy [1, 2, 3, 4, 5, 6].

A unique aspect for biologic drugs is that the immune system can recognize these molecules, leading to the formation of antibodies [7]. These anti-drug antibodies (anti-drug Abs - ADAs) impair the efficacy of the drug by either blocking the antigen-binding site or by forming complexes with the molecule, leading to an up-regulated clearance. Several analyses have implicated that low serum anti-TNF concentrations – which are variably associated with the formation of anti-drug antibodies – are associated with treatment failure [8, 9, 10], thus, the use of therapeutic drug monitoring (TDM), defined as measurement of serum drug and/or ADA concentrations, has been put forward to aid clinical decision-making for patients with IBD.

Although our therapeutic options to treat IBD is continuously evolving, the therapeutic armamentarium in IBD is still limited. Therefore, optimizing available biological treatment options including tight patient monitoring and taking advantage of TDM based optimization of patient management in patients with treatment failure should be thrived for to reach optimal long-term outcomes.

The use of TDM in anti-TNF treated patients is challenging, including interpretation the results of serum drug and ADA values and its positioning in treatment algorithms in clinical practice. This book chapter summarizes the evidence on the use of TDM during anti-TNF therapy to guide therapeutic interventions, including proactive TDM in everyday clinical practice.

Anti-TNF Drug/Anti-Drug Antibody Concentrations and Clinical Efficacy

In this section, we summarize data on anti-TNF serum concentrations, presence of ADAs and clinical outcomes. TDM has become one of the most important tools in identifying the mechanism of LOR. The existing data regarding the relationship between anti-TNF serum concentrations, ADAs and clinical outcome is limited. Most available data are retrospective. Some studies evaluated clinical efficacy only through symptom based endpoints, such as disease activity indices, which are subjective and not necessarily related to IBD. In addition, an important limitation is the heterogeneity of TDM assays including methodology differences used in the different studies, which can significantly impact these findings.

Overview of Technical Aspects of Anti-TNF Concentration and ADA Measurements

Most tests for the detection of anti-TNF concentration and ADA concentrations are based on enzyme-linked immunosorbent assay (ELISA) [11]. Radioimmunoassay (RIA) technology is also available [12]. For existing commercially available assays for antibodies, the presence of persistent drug in the serum generally interferes with the detection of ADAs, by some tests more than others [13]. All ADA assays are drug-sensitive to some extent because most assays use the drug itself as labeled detecting antibody. Various modified ELISA methods have been constructed to circumvent this problem, e.g., ELISA using anti-human λ light chain. By using the anti-human λ chain based ELISA, ADAs were detected in additional 6.3% of patients [14]. Newer assays, based on high-performance liquid chromatography (HPLC) or the pH shift-anti-idiotype method (homogenous mobility shift assay-HMSA), which can detect ADAs in the presence of circulating drug have been developed, however these methods are mainly available for infliximab (IFX) and are used less in everyday clinical practice [15, 16]. These assays also can detect antibodies with weak affinities, eliminate nonspecific binding of irrelevant IgG, and overall have increased sensitivity and specificity compared to ELISA. Since assay methodology and sensitivity differs significantly, comparisons between results obtained using different assays and/or assay techniques should be made with caution. Steenholdt et al. performed a post hoc analysis comparing the measurement of IFX serum levels and antibodies using RIA technique, ELISA, and HMSA. Authors concluded that despite differences in the techniques used among the various drug assays, the majority of cases were able to consistently identify classifications and interventions for IFX treatment failure, although comparing quantitative results is more problematic [17].

Clinical Relevance of Serum Anti-TNF Drug Concentrations

Therapeutic drug monitoring revealed important pharmacokinetic features of anti-TNF drugs. The preferred time point of sampling is the trough concentration– which means the latest time point, corresponding to the lowest concentration of drug just before the next administration. Drug trough concentrations depend on absorption, distribution, and metabolization of the drug [18]. It can be hypothesized that a trough level (TL) reflects clinical efficacy. However, TLs above a certain threshold do not necessarily result in increased efficacy. This concept is often referred to as the optimal therapeutic window concept [19]. Evidence however is conflictive, even for IFX and the optimal window concept is even more questionable for the other biologicals, e.g., optimal levels may be different during induction and maintenance therapy.

Multiple studies showed that higher IFX or adalimumab TLs were associated with higher clinical efficacy at multiple time-points and also may predict clinical outcomes in CD and UC. An analysis from ACCENT I and ACCENT II trials showed that patients with lower trough serum IFX concentrations were less likely to achieve clinical response [20, 21]. Maser et al. measured IFX trough and ADA concentrations in 105 CD patients. After a median of 14 infusions, the rate of clinical remission was higher in patients with a detectable serum IFX TL compared to patients in whom serum IFX was undetectable, including those without antibodies ($p < 0.001$). A detectable serum IFX TL was also associated with a lower C-reactive protein (CRP) (2.0 vs 11.8 mg/L; $p < 0.001$) and a higher rate of endoscopic improvement (88% vs 33%; $p < 0.001$) [8]. An observational analysis of 108

UC patients treated with scheduled IFX maintenance therapy found detectable trough IFX concentration to be a positive predictor for clinical remission and endoscopic improvement, as well [9].

In a Danish study, 106 CD patients were assessed retrospectively. IFX levels were significantly lower, and ADA levels were significantly higher in patients with LOR compared to patients in remission (median IFX TL: 0μg/mL versus 2.8μg/mL; median ADA level: 35U/mL versus 0U/mL). Optimal cut-off values were defined as IFX TL ≤0.5μg/mL, which was associated with LOR (sensitivity: 86%, specificity: 85%) and ADA ≥10U/mL (sensitivity: 81%, specificity: 90%) [22]. A more recent meta-analysis of 2,021 serum samples from 532 CD patients evaluated the correlation between infliximab concentration, ADAs, and CRP [23]. Receiver operator curve analysis showed that an IFX concentration >3 μg/ml was predictive of lower disease activity, as measured by CRP. These results are in line with data by Bortlik et al. who found that IFX TL>3 μg/ml at the beginning of maintenance treatment were predictive of sustained remission (median 2-year follow-up) in a cohort of 84 CD patients [24]. Based on published data, an IFX TL of 3-7 μg/mL during maintenance therapy correlated with sustained clinical outcomes [24, 25, 26]. In the TAXIT trial serum concentrations of ≤7 μg/ml allowed safe reduction of IFX dose [26, 27].

As for adalimumab, a similar correlation between the mean trough concentrations and clinical outcome was found during the milestone CLASSIC 1 trial but a recent post hoc analysis of both CLASSIC 1 and 2 trials was not able to determinate a reliable therapeutic cut-off value [28]. Mazor et al. identified a drug TL of 5.85 μg/mL as the optimal cut-off for predicting remission (as asymptomatic patients and normalization of CRP) [29]. In a Japanese study a TL of 5.9 μg/mL was identified to best predict normal CRP in a receiver operator curve analysis [30].

Another IgG1 monoclonal antibody is golimumab which was superior to placebo in inducing clinical response at week 6 and maintaining remission at weeks 30 and 54 in the PURSUIT trial [31, 32]. Sandborn et al. performed a phase 3, double-blind trial of 464 patients who completed golimumab induction trials. Among randomized patients on golimumab 50-mg or 100-

mg every 4 weeks, greater proportions of patients in the higher serum golimumab concentration quartiles measured at week 54 achieved clinical response through week 54 or clinical remission at both weeks 30 and 54 when compared with those in the lower serum concentration quartiles. 59% of patients in clinical remission at both weeks 30 and 54 have a golimumab TL higher than 4.27μg/mL [32].

Certolizumab pegol is another effective anti-TNF biologic as shown by Schreiber et al. in the PRECISE 2 study Certolizumab differs from other IgG1 monoclonal anti-TNFs in that it is a pegylated Fab fragment. Colombel et al. performed a post hoc analysis of the MUSIC trial to determine association between drug levels and endoscopic remission in ileocolonic CD patients [34] and found that high serum drug levels for certolizumab pegol at week 8 (range 11.1 ug/mL to 19.8 ug/mL) are associated with endoscopic response at 10 weeks and remission at 54 weeks.

New biologic drugs are also available with different mechanisms of action, which provides great comfort in cases of treatment failure to anti-TNF agents. Vedolizumab is a humanized monoclonal antibody against the a4b7 integrin inhibitor and was approved for the management of moderate to severe CD in 2014. Ustekinumab is an inhibitor of the p40 subunit of interleukins 12 and 23 and was approved for the treatment of CD in October 2016.

In conclusion, available evidence suggests that there is a relationship between anti-TNF trough serum concentrations and clinical efficacy endpoints (both objective and symptom-related) in IBD patients, although statistical significance varies.

Clinical Impact of Anti-Drug Antibodies

Immunogenicity is an important with biologic drugs. These ADAs attenuate the activity of the drug by causing faster clearance and by blocking the binding site of the drug to TNF. ADAs can also lead to allergic reactions [6, 27]

ADAs against IFX may develop up to 60% in patients on episodic therapy, causing infusion reactions, delayed serum sickness-like reactions, and may reduce the duration of patient response to treatment [35, 36]. In 105 patients with CD treated with 5 mg/kg IFX scheduled maintenance therapy, 21% of patients had detectable antibodies, 25% were antibody negative, and 54% were antibody inconclusive after a median of 14 infusions. ADA formation was associated with a higher rate of infusion reactions [8].

Baert et al. evaluated the clinical influence of ADAs in a cohort of 125 CD patients, treated with episodic IFX infusions. They concluded that presence of ADAs was independently associated with a shorter duration of response ($p < 0.001$) [35]. Low IFX TL and high ADA level was found in 10/12 patients (83%) with complete loss of response to IFX, and only in 2/24 patients (8%, $p < 0.001$) with maintained remission on scheduled IFX treatment of 62 patients tested by Ben-Horin et al. ADA status was independently associated with LOR in multivariate analysis ($p = 0.02$) [37]. In an analysis of CD patients receiving IFX, all patients (8/8) who lost response had ADAs present by fluid-phase RIA, whereas 53% (10/19) who maintained response had them, indicating that ADA presence is not always associated with lack of response. On the other hand, patients with loss of response had higher median ADA titers than patients who maintained response [12].

Adalimumab can also induce antibody formation and ADA positivity may also be the cause of LOR in adalimumab treated patients. In the CLASSIC-II maintenance study 2.8-3.7% of patients were positive for ADA during the 52-week study [38]. An association between LOR and the presence of ADAs was reported also in adalimumab treated CD patients as shown by Karamiris, et al. Antibodies against adalimumab were present in 9.2% of these patients and appeared to affect trough serum concentration [10]. In a Hungarian study involving 112 IBD patients and evaluating the frequency and predictive factors of LOR to adalimumab therapy, the cumulative ADA positivity (>10ng/mL) was 12.1% after one year and 17.3% after two years of adalimumab therapy [39]. ADA positivity was associated with LOR ($p = 0.007$ OR: 3.6 CI 95%: 1.4-9.5) [39].

In an attempt to further reduce the risk for immunogenicity, antibody derivatives were developed such as certolizumab pegol but also here an ADA response was described in 9.0% of treated CD patients [33]. Sandborn et al. evaluated the development of antibodies and effect on disease activity in certolizumab pegol treated patients, and found that median C-reactive protein and fecal calprotectin were higher ($P < 0.05$) and plasma certolizumab pegol concentrations were significantly lower ($P < 0.0001$) in patients with persistent ADAs [40].

Decreased ADA formation in patients on combined immunosuppressive therapy was reported in multiple clinical trials and cohort studies [41, 42]. Concomitant immunomodulators, including pre-infusion corticosteroids [43] azathioprine and methotrexate were reported to reduce ADA formation in patients treated with IFX [35]. In addition, concomitant immunosuppression with azathioprine was associated with superior efficacy superior compared to monotherapy with any one agent in the SONIC trial including immunosuppressive naïve early CD patients [44]. Less data is available concerning the use of combination immunosuppressive therapy with adalimumab treated patients. Kopylov et al. assessed the use of immunomodulators in adalimumab patients in a systematic review. Combination therapy with adalimumab and immunomodulator was superior to adalimumab monotherapy for induction of remission in CD ($p = 0.02$), however the rate of remission at 1 year and the need for dose escalation were similar in both groups [45].

In conclusion, available data suggest that the presence of ADAs has a potential, but not absolute, negative impact on clinical outcomes, which is probably related to altered drug clearance.

Therapeutic Drug Monitoring in Clinical Practice

Based on multiple studies, 10%-30% of patients IBD show no initial clinical benefit to anti-TNF therapy (PNR), and another 20%–50% of patients undergo secondary loss of response (sLOR) within 1 year of treatment which result in the need for dose-intensification, or discontinuation of the therapy. The annual risk of LOR seems to be comparable for IFX and adalimumab [3, 4, 5, 6].

As outlined in the previous sections, mechanisms underlining PNR and sLOR are often characterized by inadequate serum drug concentrations. Subtherapeutic or undetectable drug concentrations can arise from increased non-immune clearance of the drug, or also the increased immune-mediated clearance of the biologic. High immune clearance has been attributed to immunogenicity, and the development of ADAs resulting in high immune clearance of the anti-TNF drug. Immunogenicity may also result in drug intolerance and treatment failure through the occurrence of infusion reactions [3, 4, 13, 35, 37, 46].

As earlier discussed, numerous pivotal studies suggest a positive correlation between high serum drug concentrations and favorable therapeutic outcomes including clinical, biomarker and endoscopic remission, whereas ADAs have been associated with sLOR and infusion reactions [8, 9, 10, 20, 21, 22, 23, 27, 28, 29, 30, 35, 37]. As objective outcome parameters are emerging as new therapeutic goals in IBD [47], this correlation carries a great clinical importance and supports the concept of frequent TDM, comprising the measurement of serum drug levels and anti-drug antibodies in IBD clinical practice.

After the initiation of anti-TNF therapy in patients, primarily three different strategies/clinical scenarios have been proposed so far that may require TDM-based management. These scenarios are anti-TNF treatment failure and its prevention, and discontinuation of anti-TNF therapy during remission [48].

However, implementing TDM in real-life clinical practice poses challenges and is limited by the heterogeneity in study design, therapeutic outcomes and assays used, interpretation of serum drug and/or ADA assay values, which have hindered the identification of clinically relevant standard concentration thresholds [48]. Validation of a treatment algorithm using TDM in clinical practice also needs more extensive research. This chapter will focus mainly on the role of TDM in clinical practice and guiding therapeutic decisions in IBD as we stand nowadays.

Interpreting the Results of TDM – Cut-off Values of Trough Levels and Anti-Drug Antibodies

Based on recently published data, studies suggest that the optimal therapeutic drug trough concentration during maintenance therapy is 3-7 μg/ml for IFX and 5-10 μg/ml for adalimumab [22, 23, 25, 26, 27, 29, 30]. The choice of therapeutic threshold drug TL concentration is critical when evaluating patients who lose response to therapy and to guide treatment decisions. It is important to note that target trough concentration is not a sole value rather a range of values and may vary by treatment target (clinical remission vs endoscopic remission), disease state (high disease activity vs low disease activity), or phase of therapy (induction vs maintenance). Vande Casteele et al. evaluated 6 studies on IFX and 6 studies on adalimumab also in a recent review to examine potential trough concentration thresholds [49]. Taken together these results, they evaluated the relative proportion of patients who were or were not in remission, above and below a target TL. These data were derived largely from cross-sectional studies of maintenance therapy, where authors reported the sensitivity and specificity of concentration thresholds in predicting the presence of clinical remission (or response). Data on the relative performance of different IFX TL thresholds derived from 6 studies is presented in Table 1 [50, 51, 52, 53, 54, 55]. The proportion of patients not in clinical remission above IFX trough concentration thresholds decreases with increasing trough concentration. The probability of not being in clinical remission is low if IFX TL is 7 μg/mL or more during maintenance therapy [49]. Results on TL thresholds for adalimumab maintenance therapy are presented in Table 2, of note less potential cut-off values were studied [56, 57, 58, 59, 60, 61]. For certolizumab pegol maintenance therapy, we included data from a large exposure-response pooled analysis, including data from 9 trials encompassing 2157 patients. Table 3 [62].

Table 1. Distribution of patients according to clinical status, at different infliximab cut-offs in cross-sectional or cohort studies [49]

Infliximab	**Trough at or above cut-off**
cut-off, µg/mL	Patients not in remission, % (95% CI)
1	24.8 (17.7-33.7)
3	14.7 (9.7-21.7)
5	7.9 (4.6-13.2)
7	3.9 (1.5-9.5)
10	4.3 (1.8-9.6)

Table 2. Distribution of patients according to clinical status, at different adalimumab cut-offs in cross-sectional or cohort studies [49]

Adalimumab	**Trough at or above cut-off**
cut-off, µg/mL	Patients not in remission, % (95% CI)
5.0 ± 1	17.0 (12.7-22.5)
7.5 ± 1	10.3 (6.1-16.9)

Table 3. Distribution of patients according to clinical status, at different certolizumab pegol cut-offs (pooled analysis of individual participant data of 9 trials) [49, 62]

Adalimumab	**Trough at or above cut-off**
cut-off, µg/mL	Patients not in remission, % (95% CI)
10	41.6
15	32.2
20	25.5

Considering objective outcomes, like mucosal healing, different TL cut-off values have been reported. Ungar et al. performed a retrospective cross-sectional analysis of 145 patients with IBD treated with IFX (n = 78) or adalimumab (n = 67) at a medical center in Israel to determine drug levels associated with mucosal healing in IBD patients. Increasing levels of IFX beyond 8 µg/mL produced only minimal increases in the rate of mucosal healing, whereas the association between higher level of adalimumab and increased rate of mucosal healing reached a plateau at 12 μg/mL. Authors proposed that serum levels of 6–10 μg/mL for IFX and 8–12 μg/mL for adalimumab are required to achieve mucosal healing in 80%–90% of patients with IBD, and that this could be considered as a "therapeutic window" [63].

There is little information on drug TL cut-offs during induction therapy. Values vary greatly depending on time of sampling and target outcomes. Adedokun et al. proposed a cut-off of 22.0 μg/mL at week 6 for IFX, which was associated with clinical response at week 8. Thresholds of 5.1 μg/mL and 3.7 μg/mL, were predictive of clinical response at week 14 and week 30, respectively [64]. In a prospective, multicenter study, the predictive potential of TDM on short- and medium-term efficacy of biosimilar IFX therapy was evaluated in Hungary, involving a total of 291 consecutive IBD patients. In UC patients, TLs at Week 2 predicted both clinical response and remission at Weeks 14 and 30 (clinical remission at Week 14: area under the curve [AUC] = 0.79, cut-off: 15.3μg/ml; remission at Week 30: AUC = 0.74, cut-off: 14.5 μg/ml). Similarly, TLs at Week 2 predicted short-term clinical efficacy in CD patients. In addition, early ADA status by Week 14 was associated with short-and medium-term clinical response and remission [65]. During adalimumab induction therapy, a week 4 cut-off of >11.0 μg/mL was best predictive for clinical remission at week 12, as proposed by Vande Casteele et al. [66].

In contrast to trough concentrations, quantitative results of ADAs from different assays are much more difficult to compare, and should be interpreted qualitatively in the appropriate clinical context. Correlations between established assays are lacking, and assay-related variability is considerable. In a cohort study of 125 patients with CD by Baert et al, an ADA concentration of >8 μg/mL was considered "high" and correlated with a shorter duration of response [35]. In the retrospective study of Yanai et al, a threshold for ADAs to IFX of >9 μg/mL equivalent and for ADAs to adalimumab of >4 μg/mL was proposed that identified patients with high ADAs who did not respond to empiric dose escalation with 90% specificity [67]. In a Hungarian study by Gonczi et al. a different assay was used for adalimumab (Lisa Tracker, Theradiag, France). Authors defined high ADA titres as >200ng/ml to better stratify patients. The cut-off value of detectable ADA levels by the assay used was 10 ng/ml. Rate of low TL in patients with high ADA was 85.7%, while it was 28.6% in patients with low ADA and 27.5% in ADA negative patients ($p = 0.006$; $p = 0{,}004$). LOR was associated with ADA positivity, even if patients with low or high titre ADA were analyzed separately ($p = 0.039$) [39].

In summary, optimal target trough concentrations and timing of achieving maximal effectiveness of anti-TNF agents during induction and maintenance therapy are still unclear. The studies used to derive different target TLs were mainly cross-sectional studies of patients on maintenance therapy and they were not specifically designed to evaluate patients who had a secondary loss of response. Based on the currently available evidence, the American Gastroenterological Association (AGA) panel suggests target trough concentrations of 5 mg/mL for IFX, 7.5 mg/mL for adalimumab, and 20 mg/L for certolizumab pegol, to guide treatment decision in patients who are experiencing secondary loss of response on maintenance therapy [68].

Management of Anti-TNF Treatment Failure by TDM Based Strategies

Current guidelines and clinical practice suggest intensifying the anti-TNF treatment regimen in case of secondary treatment failure [69, 70]. This ‘empiric’ strategy is based on the assumption that it is preferable to completely exhaust treatment options with the current anti-TNF agent before discontinuing its use. These strategies are based on uncontrolled observations from clinical trials and cohort studies showing that clinical effect can be restored in the short term in more than half of the patients [3, 4, 6]. However, a substantial proportion of patients does not respond to anti-TNF treatment intensification or loses response to the intensified regimen over time ultimately leading to complete treatment failure and discontinuation of the drug. Switching to a different TNF-inhibitor within drug class is generally preferred in this scenario and the overall rate of recapturing response is similar to that of the dose intensification with the primary anti-TNF. Of note, long term efficacy is decreased as compared with the primary anti-TNF agent [71, 72, 73, 74]. Switching out of class to another biologic agent with different mode of action has recently become an alternative by the approval of vedolizumab and ustekinumab.

The empiric approach of managing loss of response is considered frequently suboptimal and may lead to additional costs. The TDM-based strategy by applying measurements of anti-TNF drug levels and anti-drug antibodies at the time of manifest treatment failure offers an alternative. The goal of TDM at treatment failure is to identify the potential underlying pharmacokinetic (PK) and pharmacodynamic (PD) related mechanisms responsible for the lack of the desired effect in each individual patient, and to guide clinical interventions accordingly.

The TDM based therapeutic strategy has several advantages over the empiric approach. First, it could help avoiding dose intensification in those patients who will not benefit from increased dosage of the drug (i.e., patients with increased immune-mediated clearance of the drug or patients who have a non-TNF driven disease or other causes of symptoms), (2) in those patients who lost response due to low concentrations of drug, TDM allows targeted dose intensification, and (3) directs patients to other now available therapeutic options when appropriate [46, 48].

At present, TDM is most commonly used in clinical practice in case of suspicion of active disease and sLOR. In the past few years, numerous studies investigated and showed the utility of serum anti-TNF TL and ADA level measurements in the management of sLOR, regarding both infliximab and adalimumab [27, 45, 67, 75, 76, 77, 78, 79]. These studies proposed that patients with subtherapeutic drug levels, but negative or low levels of ADA will benefit more from dose escalation compared with switching to another anti-TNF. Those with adequate drug levels are likely to respond better to changing to a biological agent with a different mechanism of action, as disease activity and inflammation in these patients may not respond to anti-TNF (non-immune mediated reasons for anti-TNF treatment failure). Moreover, studies demonstrated that patients who lose response to anti-TNF therapy due to ADA responded well when switched to another anti-TNF agent. Although, those with transient and/or low titre ADA may still benefit from optimization of original anti-TNF therapy. Some recommend switching between anti-TNF agents at loss of response only at high-titre ADAs and sub-therapeutic drug levels, since ADAs are sometimes only transient without a clinical impact. Dose intensification combined with optimized immunosuppressive therapy at low-titre ADAs may be beneficial in a proportion of patients [80, 81, 82]. Yanai et al. showed that patients with high titers of ADAs had longer durations of response when anti-TNF agents were switched than when dosage was increased ($p = 0.03$; log-rank test), although dosage increases were more effective for patients with no or low titers of ADAs ($p = 0.02$) [67]. A recent retrospective study including 90 IBD patients treated with infliximab revealed that antibodies classified as 'transient' (patient tested positive for ADA during follow-up on at least one time point and negative on the next measurement) led to a discontinuation of the treatment in only 13% of the patients as compared to 68% of the patients who developed 'sustained antibodies' [83]. In a study published from the Mayo clinic [77], authors measured TLs and the presence of ADAs in 155 patients. In patients with subtherapeutic IFX concentrations, dose escalation was associated with a clinical response in 86%, compared to a 33% in patients changing to another anti-TNF. However, in patients with ADA positivity, change to another anti-TNF agent was associated with a response in 92%, whereas dose escalation had a response of only 17%. Similar results were published more recently from Israel and France [67, 78]. A retrospective study of 64 CD patients and 26 UC patients showed significantly lower response rates after IFX dose intensification in the presence of persistent anti-IFX antibodies (16%) as compared to dose intensification in patients with transient anti-IFX antibodies (69%) or without anti-IFX antibodies (94%) [83].

Similar conclusions resulted from studies evaluating LOR in adalimumab therapy. Roblin et al. conducted a prospective observational study where 82 IBD patients on adalimumab with sLOR were first dose intensified on adalimumab and followed by switching to IFX in the absence of response [78]. Patients were divided into three groups based on adalimumab trough levels and based on previous studies: group A, adalimumab TL >4.9 μg/ml; group B, adalimumab TL < 4.9 μg/ml and undetectable levels of ADA (< 10 ng/ml); and group C, adalimumab TL < 4.9 μg/ml and ADA >10 ng/ml. Patients with insufficient adalimumab levels without ADAs had significantly higher remission rates on an intensified adalimumab regimen (67%) as compared to patients with detectable antibodies (12%). Clinical remission rates following IFX initiation were 6.9%, 25%, and 80% in groups A, B, and C, respectively, and duration of response to IFX was also significantly higher in group C [78].

Steenholdt et al. conducted a randomized controlled trial (RCT) in Denmark designed to compare empiric anti-TNF treatment intensification and personalized TDM-based strategies at anti-TNF treatment failure and to investigate the cost-effectiveness of interventions based on TDM. In this multicenter study, 69 CD patients with symptomatic treatment failure to IFX during standard maintenance therapy were equally randomized to IFX dose intensification (5 mg/kg every 4 weeks) or interventions based on serum IFX TL and ADA levels using the proposed algorithm. After 12 weeks, clinical response rates were comparable between the two strategies (53% vs. 58%), which indicates that the TDM-based strategy did not result in inferior efficacy compared with empiric dose intensification. Costs were substantially lower (34% reduction) for those treated in accordance with the algorithm than by empiric IFX dose intensification, which was attained by avoiding inappropriate dose escalations [75, 76]. In a simulation model study, TDM-based interventions have also shown to be more cost effective compared to empiric dose escalations in patients at sLOR, while similar clinical outcomes were achieved [84].

Similar findings supporting clinical non-inferiority of TDM-based strategies compared with empiric treatment at adalimumab treatment failure has also been reported [59].

Based on the same studies we discussed above, multiple TDM-based management algorithms have been proposed for with the management of anti-TNF treatment failure. There are slight differences in details among these algorithms, primarily related to the timing and method of objective disease activity assessment prior to measuring TLs and ADA levels [27, 77, 78, 79]. However, the key recommendations at sLOR regarding the clinical scenarios of different combinations of TL and ADA level results at TDM are consistent. The suggested therapeutic algorithm for the optimal management of anti-TNF treatment failure based on TDM results is summarized in Table 4. It is important to perform an objective disease activity assessment preceding the TDM measurements. The optimal means of objective assessment (e.g., biomarkers only or additional endoscopy/cross sectional imaging) before or together with TDM assessment are yet to be determined. According to the algorithm by Ben-Horin and Chowers, symptomatic patients routinely undergo endoscopy. The TDM-based care pathway is compared to endoscopic findings in addition to clinical response [73]. In contrast, Afif et al. from the Mayo Clinic and Velayos et al. from California both proposed an algorithm that restricts endoscopy to patients with symptoms in the setting of therapeutic IFX levels [77, 84]. This approach sets a balance between making decisions on the basis of objective data and the efficient use of resources. Based on serum and faecal inflammatory biomarker testing, patients with evidence of active disease undergo TDM to determine the most appropriate therapeutic option. Only patients with specific indications undergo endoscopic or cross-sectional imaging.

The considerations regarding TDM-based clinical interventions in patients with secondary treatment failure are in principle similar in patients presenting with primary anti-TNF treatment failure. However, data considering this subgroup is almost non-existing and special conditions regarding increased drug clearance among these patients may apply [85]. Of note the value of TDM assessment in overt PNR is limited in the everyday practice, especially in patients with severe clinical activity.

In summary, available evidence appears to support a TDM-based management approach in patients presenting with manifest secondary anti-TNF treatment failure. The TDM-based strategy has several advantages over an empiric management as it avoids unnecessary dose intensification, allows targeted switch between anti-TNF agents, and if appropriate, directs therapy to other now available therapeutic options. Clinical outcomes were not found superior, but were achieved at reduced costs.

Table 4. TDM-based treatment algorithm for handling patients with anti-TNF treatment failure [48, 77]

	IBD patients at treatment failure →	Confirm inflammation: • Biomarkers (CRP, FC) (endoscopy/imaging) • Verify drug adherence • Exclude IBS, infections, malignancy, strictures, etc.
	Detectable anti-drug Abs	***Undetectable anti-drug Abs***
Sub-therapeutic anti-TNF drug levels	Insufficient bioavailability of the anti-TNF agent due to induced immunogenicity with functional anti-drug Abs that increase drug clearance. ↓ **Change to different TNF-inhibitor.**	Insufficient anti-TNF drug bioavailability due to non-immune mediated pharmacokinetic issues. Alternatively, potential compliance issues. ↓ **Intensify the treatment regimen of the currently used TNF-inhibitor.**
Therapeutic anti-TNF drug levels	Non-functional anti-drug Abs. **or** False positive anti-drug Abs test. ↓ Repeat assessments of anti-TNF drug and anti-drug Abs over time. Review of clinical condition: If symptoms are caused by IBD related inflammation, **switch to another biological agent with a different mechanism of action.**	Pharmacodynamic issues where inhibition of TNF-α is ineffective due to non-TNF driven disease. **or** Symptoms caused by other problems than active IBD. ↓ TNF-inhibitors are not effective and to be discontinued. Review of clinical condition: If symptoms are caused by IBD related inflammation, **switch to another biological agent with a different mechanism of action.**

Prevention of Anti-TNF Treatment Failure by TDM Based Strategies - Role of Proactive TDM Measurement in Clinical Practice

In addition to helping the clinical management of patients with manifest anti-TNF treatment failure, TDM-based strategies have also been proposed to prevent treatment failure among patients with stable clinical responses on anti-TNF maintenance treatment [86, 87, 88]. The hypothesis is based on findings that low anti-TNF serum drug level is associated with low efficacy and/or treatment failure during maintenance or induction [9, 31, 89, 90]. Based on these results, one could hypothesize that disease control could be reached by proactive dose optimization of patients based on serial TDM measurements, by maintaining drug levels in the therapeutic window [91]. Conversely, drug concentrations above the therapeutic window will not result in increased efficacy, and dose can be de-escalated in patients with supra-therapeutic drug levels to save costs [20, 21, 22, 23, 92, 93]. Of note, high anti-TNF drug concentrations were not associated with unfavorable safety signal, however association between skin lesions, arthralgia and very high anti-TNF TLs have been suggested [94].

The first observational study published to demonstrate the efficacy of proactive TDM-based dose optimization included 126 patients with IBD. In this study, patients in clinical remission who underwent proactive TDM and IFX dose optimization targeting a therapeutic window of 5–10 µg/mL had markedly improved infliximab sustainability when compared with control patients on reactive TDM or empiric dose escalation only [95].

The landmark Trough level Adapted infliXImab Treatment (TAXIT) trial, an RCT enrolling 263 IBD patients with stable clinical responses investigated if dosing of IFX based on trough levels measured prior to each infusion and adjusted accordingly by proactive TDM was superior compared to clinically based dosing of IFX [26]. The study was comprised of two phases. In the first phase of this study, all patients were dose optimized to IFX trough levels of 3-7 µg/mL. This intervention resulted in a significant drop in HBI index and CRP and a higher proportion of patients in clinical remission (65% vs. 88%) in the subgroup with initially suboptimal IFX levels of <3 μg/mL. In contrast, patients with IFX levels >7 μg/mL had successful dose de-escalation without affecting remission rates, but with a reduction of drug costs of 28%. In the second phase of the study, patients were randomized 1:1 to continued treatment according to the proactive TDM-based strategy or, to switch back to clinically based dosing. However, the primary end-point of the study, clinical and biochemical remission at one year after optimization was similar in both groups (69% vs. 66%). Consequently, the study showed no additional benefit in utilizing an ongoing proactive TDM-based strategy to clinically-based dosing after the initial optimization phase. However, the group applying the proactive TDM-based strategy had significantly fewer disease flares needing rescue therapy (7% vs. 17%), and less frequent undetectable IFX trough levels. Of note, while patients with concentrations of >7 μg/mL allowed safe dose reduction, resulting in cost savings, the overall difference in costs between the two different strategies was small [26].

There are only limited data regarding the role of TDM during anti-TNF induction therapy. Nevertheless, higher infliximab concentrations during and early after the induction phase are associated with favorable short-term and long-term therapeutic outcomes, whereas low or undetectable drug concentrations and ADA are associated with PNR, sLOR and drug discontinuation [56, 89, 96]. These observations would suggest that target concentration adjusted dosing should be implement early on, possibly even during the induction therapy. TAILORIX [97] is a prospective RCT examining early proactive TDM-based IFX optimization applied after the induction phase. Biologic naïve adult patients with active CD received induction treatment with 3 infusions of IFX 5 mg/kg in combination with immunosuppressants. At week 14, patients were randomized to 1 of 3 different maintenance strategies: 1) dose intensification of IFX in steps of 2,5 mg/kg based on clinical symptoms, biomarker analysis and serum IFX concentrations drawn before the previous infusion; 2) dose intensification of IFX from 5 to 10 mg/kg based on the same criteria; and 3) IFX dose increase to 10 mg/kg based on clinical symptoms alone. The primary endpoint of the trial was sustained steroid-free clinical remission from week 22 to 54 and absence of ulceration on endoscopy at 1 year. Target for IFX dosing was a trough concentration > 3 ug/ml. The proportions of patients without ulcerations at week 54 were 36%, 43%, and 48% (p = NS) and with endoscopic remission (CDEIS < 3) 49%, 51%, and 45% (p = NS). According to the results, proactive trough level–based dose intensification was not superior to dose intensification based on clinical symptoms alone in patients with active CD [97].

In summary, the TAXIT and TAILORIX studies show no additional value of routine ongoing/proactive TDM during maintenance therapy as measured by medium term clinical activity or endoscopic activity as outcome. However, these findings indicate that there might be a benefit to a subset of presumably under-dosed patients for conducting one-time proactive TDM to optimize IFX therapy during maintenance phase. More data on the utility of proactive TDM strategy are needed. For example, an optimal concentration therapeutic window, the clinically most relevant time point of measuring drug concentrations and the most suitable assay to be used are still waiting to be clearly determined. Studies should also assess the overall cost-effectiveness by taking into account expenses for repeated measurements of drug and anti-drug Abs and dose escalation in patients with proposed sub-therapeutic drug levels.

Discontinuation of Anti-TNF Therapy during Remission Based on TDM Strategies

Discontinuation of anti-TNF therapy can be considered for multiple reasons such as high costs of therapy or patient's preferences, including beliefs on increased risk of infectious complications or malignancies [98, 99, 100]. Current guidelines provide no recommendations with respect to stopping anti-TNF therapies, and decision is typically based on an estimated, case-by-case, benefit-risk ratio considering individual patients.

Evidence regarding CD comes from the landmark STORI trial and a few retrospective observational studies. Approximately 50% of patients with Crohn's disease who were treated for at least 1 year with IFX combined with an immunosuppressive agent experienced a relapse within 1 year after discontinuation of IFX. However, it was possible to identify a subgroup of patients with a considerably lower risk of relapse using a combination of clinical and biologic markers (absence of surgical resection, leukocyte counts >6.0 × 10(9)/L, and levels of hemoglobin ≤145 g/L, C-reactive protein ≥5.0 mg/L, and fecal calprotectin ≥300 μg/g) [101]. Steenholdt et al, and some other uncontrolled observations of patients having discontinued IFX therapy while in clinical remission, have reported app. half of patients to maintain remission after one year. However, a subgroup of up to one third of patients presumably characterized by clinical, biochemical, and endoscopical remission seem to have a long-lasting favorable prognosis without relapse after discontinuation of IFX therapy [102, 103, 104, 105]. Fifty-one UC and 121 CD patients who had achieved clinical remission following 1 year of infliximab therapy and for whom infliximab was then discontinued were included in a Hungarian prospective study by Molnar et al. [106, 107]. Results showed, that 35% and 45% of UC/CD patients needed to be retreated with infliximab within 1 year after treatment cessation. Previous biological therapy and was associated with the need for restarting biological therapy both in UC and CD ($p = 0.021$; $p = 0.011$). Whether these results are because interruption of IFX have coincided with the naturally occurring phase of disease quiescence, or anti-TNF therapy changes the natural course of IBD still remains debated. Drobne et al. performed a retrospective study to determine the effect of immune-suppressant withdrawal on biologic drug levels [108]. A total of 117 patients had adequate disease control and immunosuppressant drug was withdrawn with biologic serum levels drawn before and after withdrawal. The study showed that 38% of patients required dose escalation and 18% required discontinuation of biologic therapy. High (>5 μg/mL) infliximab trough levels at the time of immunomodulator withdrawal were associated with a decreased risk for infliximab dose escalation ($p = 0.03$).

The optimal anti-TNF withdrawal strategy including time spent in remission before stopping, and the optimal treatment following its discontinuation, has yet to be clearly defined. Of note, patients in remission who have undetectable IFX levels at time of discontinuation have also favorable outcomes [109, 110]. These suggest that anti-TNF discontinuation among patients in complete clinical, biochemical, and endoscopical remission may be favorably supported by a TDM-based strategy.

Conclusion

Anti-TNF drugs are important components of the therapeutic armamentarium in IBD management, yet a significant proportion of patients does not respond or lose response to treatment. Numerous studies have demonstrated a positive correlation between adequate serum anti-TNF concentrations and favorable therapeutic outcomes including clinical and endoscopic remission, whereas ADA have been associated with secondary LOR and infusion reactions. This book chapter summarized the use of TDM based algorithms in the clinical practice to achieve personalized treatment with TNF inhibitors. Currently, evidence supports the use of TDM at failure of therapy. TDM-based treatment algorithms are proposed to guide interventions to reach optimal clinical, economic, and patient reported outcomes.

TDM-based strategies may prevent anti-TNF treatment failure during ongoing therapy by routine TL and ADA measurements. However, in clinical trials, in patients on long-standing biological therapy, serial monitoring of drug concentrations has no additional benefit compared to clinically-based strategy and is equally effective after one-year of therapy. In addition, observations suggest that anti-TNF drug withdrawal during remission may be achievable in selected subgroups, supporting a novel use of TDM to support decisions at drug withdrawal.

However, there are still challenges regarding the application of a TDM-guided treatment strategy. Despite emerging data, the 'therapeutic window' concept of anti-TNFs, including suggested cut-offs at certain treatment scenarios, as well as clinical implications of positive ADA testing (interpretations of ADA levels, considering that low- or high-ADA titres and transient vs. persistent ADAs are conflictive in some patients) are sometimes ambiguous. Finally, assay-related factors should be considered, including limitations and strengths.

Future research is warranted to refine personalized treatment strategies in IBD applying personalized TDM-based treatment algorithms preferably combined with relevant patient-, disease-, and treatment related characteristics integrated into a single complex model.

REFERENCES

[1] Hanauer SB, Feagan BG, Lichtenstein GR, et al. Maintenance infliximab for Crohn's disease: the ACCENT I randomised trial. *Lancet.* 2002;359:1541-9.

[2] Colombel JF, Sandborn WJ, Rutgeerts P, et al. Adalimumab for maintenance of clinical response and remission in patients with Crohn's disease: the CHARM trial. *Gastroenterology.* 2007;132:52-65.

[3] Gisbert JP, Panes J. Loss of response and requirement of infliximab dose intensification in Crohn's disease: a review. *Am J Gastroenterol. 2009*;104(3):760–7.

[4] Billioud V, Sandborn WJ, Peyrin-Biroulet L. Loss of response and need for adalimumab dose intensification in Crohn's disease: a systematic review. *Am J Gastroenterol.* 2011;106(4):674–84.

[5] Schnitzler F, Fidder H, Ferrante M, et al. Long-term outcome of treatment with infliximab in 614 patients with Crohn's disease: results from a single-centre cohort. *Gut.* 2009;58(4):492–500.

[6] Ben-Horin S, Chowers Y. Review article: loss of response to anti-TNF treatments in Crohn's disease. *Aliment Pharmacol Ther* 2011;33:987–95.

[7] Schellekens H, Casadevall N. Immunogenicity of recombinant human proteins: causes and consequences. *J Neurol* 2004;251(Suppl 2):II4–II9.

[8] Maser EA, Villela R, Silverberg MS, et al. Association of trough serum Infliximab to clinical outcome after scheduled maintenance treatment for Crohn's disease. *Clin Gastroenterol Hepatol.* 2006;4(10):1248–54.

[9] Seow CH, Newman A, Irwin SP, et al. Trough serum infliximab: a predictive factor of clinical outcome for infliximab treatment in acute ulcerative colitis. *Gut.* 2010;59(1):49–54.

[10] Karmiris K, Paintaud G, Noman M, et al. Influence of trough serum levels and immunogenicity on long-term outcome of adalimumab therapy in Crohn's disease. *Gastroenterology.* 2009;137(5):1628–40.

[11] Bendtzen K, Ainsworth M, Steenholdt C, et al. Individual medicine in inflammatory bowel disease: monitoring bioavailability, pharmacokinetics and immunogenicity of anti-tumour necrosis factor-alpha antibodies. *Scand J Gastroenterol.* 2009;44:774–781.

[12] Ainsworth MA, Bendtzen K, Brynskov J. Tumor necrosis factor-alpha binding capacity and anti-infliximab antibodies measured by fluid phase radioimmunoassays as predictors of clinical efficacy of infliximab in Crohn's disease. *Am J Gastroenterol.* 2008;103:944–948.

[13] Cassinotti A, Travis S. Incidence and significance of immunogenicity to infliximab in Crohn's disease: a critical systematic review. *Inflamm Bowel Dis.* 2009;15:1264–1275.

[14] Kopylov U, Mazor Y, Yavzori M, et al. Clinical utility of antihuman lambda chain-based enzyme-linked immunosorbent assay (ELISA) versus double antigen ELISA for the detection of anti-infliximab antibodies. *Inflamm Bowel Dis.* 2012;18:1628-33.

[15] Wang S, Ohrmund L, Ling N, et al. Analysis of anti-drug antibodies (ADA) to adalimumab in patient serum using a novel homogeneous mobility shift assay. *Am J Gastroenterol.* 2010;105(suppl 1):S444–S445.

[16] Van Schouwenburg, Van Schouwenburg P, Bartelds G, et al. A novel method for the detection of antibodies to adalimumab in the presence of drug reveals ''hidden'' immunogenicity in rheumatoid arthritis. *J Immunol Methods.* 2010;362:82–88.

[17] Steenholdt C, Bendtzen K, Brynskov J, et al. Clinical implications of measuring drug and anti-drug antibodies by different assays when optimizing infliximab treatment failure in crohn's disease: Post hoc analysis of a randomized controlled trial. *Am J Gastroenterol* 2014;109(7):1055-64.

[18] Lobo ED, Hansen RJ, Balthasar JP. Antibody pharmacokinetics and pharmacodynamics. *J Pharm Sci.* 2004;93(11):2645–68.

[19] Nestorov I. Clinical pharmacokinetics of tumor necrosis factor antagonists. *J Rheumatol Suppl.* 2005;74:13–8.

[20] Fasanmade A, Olson A, Bag W, et al. Relationship between infliximab pharmacokinetics and improvement in Crohn's disease. *Gastroenterology*. 2002;122(suppl 4):A617–A618.

[21] Fasanmade AA, Marsters P, Munsanje E, et al. Infliximab pharmacokinetics and improvement in fistulizing Crohn's disease. *Gastroenterology*. 2003;124(4 suppl 1):A61.

[22] Steenholdt C, Bendtzen K, Brynskov J, et al. Cut-off levels and diagnostic accuracy of infliximab trough levels and anti-infliximab antibodies in Crohn's disease. *Scand J Gastroenterol.* 2011;46: 310-8.

[23] Feagan BG, Singh S, Lockton S, et al. 565 Novel Infliximab (IFX) and Antibody-to-Infliximab (ATI) Assays are Predictive of Disease Activity in Patients With Crohn's Disease (CD). *Gastroenterology*. 2012;142(5):S-114.

[24] Bortlik M, Duricova D, Malickova K, et al. Infliximab trough levels may predict sustained response to infliximab in patients with Crohn's disease. *J Crohns Colitis*. 2013;7(9):736–43.

[25] Vande Casteele N, Khanna R, Levesque BG et al. The relationship between infliximab concentrations, antibodies to infliximab and disease activity in Crohn's disease. *Gut.* 2015 Oct;64(10):1539-45.

[26] Vande Casteele N, Ferrante M, Van Assche G et al. Trough Concentrations of Infliximab Guide Dosing for Patients with Inflammatory Bowel Disease. *Gastroenterology* 2015;148:1320-1329.

[27] Ben-Horin S, Chowers Y. Tailoring anti-TNF therapy in IBD: drug levels and disease activity. *Nat Rev Gastroenterol Hepatol* 2014;11:243-255.

[28] Chiu YL, Rubin DT, Vermeire S, et al. Serum adalimumab concentration and clinical remission in patients with Crohn's disease. *Inflamm Bowel Dis.* 2013;19(6):1112–22. Post hoc analysis of CLASSIC 1 and CLASSIC 2 trials investigating the correlation between adalimumab trough concentration and clinical remission.

[29] Mazor Y, Almog R, Kopylov U, et al. Adalimumab drug and antibody levels as predictors of clinical and laboratory response in patients with Crohn's disease. *Aliment Pharmacol Ther*. 2014; 40(6): 620-628.

[30] Imaeda H, Takahashi K, Fujimoto T, et al. Clinical utility of newly developed immunoassays for serum concentrations of adalimumab and anti-adalimumab antibodies in patients with Crohn's disease. *J Gastroenterol.* 2014;49(1):100–9.

[31] Sandborn WJ, Feagan BG, Marano C, et al. Subcutaneous golimumab induces clinical response and remission in patients with moderate-to-severe ulcerative colitis. *Gastroenterology.* 2014 Jan;146(1):85-95.

[32] Sandborn WJ, Feagan BG, Marano C, et al. Subcutaneous golimumab maintains clinical response in patients with moderate-to severe ulcerative colitis. *Gastroenterology.* 2014;146(96–109):e1.

[33] Schreiber S, Khaliq-Kareemi M, Lawrance IC et al. Maintenance therapy with certolizumab pegol for Crohn's disease. *N Engl J Med.* 2007 Jul 19;357(3):239-50.

[34] Colombel JF, Sandborn WJ, Allez M, et al. Association between plasma concentrations of certolizumab pegol and endoscopic outcomes of patients with crohn's disease. *Clin Gastroenterol Hepatol* 2014;12:423-431.e1.

[35] Baert F, Noman M, Vermeire S, et al. Influence of immunogenicity on the long-term efficacy of infliximab in Crohn's disease. *N Engl J Med.* 2003;348:601-8.

[36] Rutgeerts P, Feagan BG, Lichtenstein GR, et al. Comparison of scheduled and episodic treatment strategies of infliximab in Crohn's disease. *Gastroenterology.* 2004;126:402-13.

[37] Ben-Horin S, Yavzori M, Katz L, et al. The immunogenic part of infliximab is the F(ab')2, but measuring antibodies to the intact infliximab molecule is more clinically useful. *Gut.* 2011;60:41-48.

[38] Sandborn W, Hanauer S, Rutgeerts P, et al. Adalimumab for maintenance treatment of Crohn's disease: results of the CLASSIC II trial. *Gut.* 2007;56:1232–1239.

[39] Gonczi L, Kurti Z, Rutka M et al. Drug persistence and need for dose intensification to adalimumab therapy; the importance of therapeutic drug monitoring in inflammatory bowel diseases. *BMC Gastroenterol.* 2017 Aug 8;17(1):97.

[40] Sandborn WJ, Wolf DC, Kosutic G, et al. Effects of transient and persistent anti-drug antibodies to certolizumab pegol. *Inflamm Bowel Dis* 2017;23:1047-1056.

[41] Vermeire S, Noman M, Van Assche G, et al. Effectiveness of concomitant immunosuppressive therapy in suppressing the formation of antibodies to infliximab in Crohn's disease. *Gut.* 2007;56:1226-31.

[42] Van Assche G, Magdelaine-Beuzelin C, Haens G, et al. Withdrawal of immunosuppression in Crohn's disease treated with scheduled infliximab maintenance: a randomized trial. *Gastroenterology.* 2008;134:1861-8.

[43] Farrell RJ, Alsahli M, Jeen YT, et al. Intravenous hydrocortisone premedication reduces antibodies to infliximab in Crohn's disease: a randomized controlled trial. *Gastroenterology.* 2003;124:917-24.

[44] Colombel JF, Sandborn WJ, Reinisch W, et al. Infliximab, azathioprine, or combination therapy for Crohn's disease. *N Engl J Med.* 2010;362:1383-95.

[45] Kopylov U, Al-Taweel T, Yaghoobi M et al. Adalimumab monotherapy versus combination therapy with immunomodulators in patients with Crohn's disease: a systematic review and meta-analysis. *J Crohns Colitis*. 2014 Dec;8(12):1632-41.

[46] Colombel JF, Feagan BG, Sandborn WJ, Van AG, Robinson AM. Therapeutic drug monitoring of biologics for inflammatory bowel disease. *Inflamm Bowel Dis* 2012; 18: 349–58.

[47] Peyrin-Biroulet L, Sandborn W, Sands BE, et al. Selecting Therapeutic Targets in Inflammatory Bowel Disease (STRIDE): Determining Therapeutic Goals for Treat-to-Target. *Am J Gastroenterol.* 2015 Sep;110(9):1324-38.

[48] Casper Steenholdt. Personalized therapy with TNF-inhibitors in Crohn's disease: Optimizing treatment outcomes by monitoring drug levels and anti-drug antibodies, *Dan Med J* 2016;63(8):B5270.

[49] Vande Casteele N, Herfarth H, Katz J et al. American Gastroenterological Association Institute Technical Review on the Role of Therapeutic Drug Monitoring in the Management of Inflammatory Bowel Diseases. *Gastroenterology.* 2017 Sep;153(3):835-857.e6. Epub 2017 Jul 31.

[50] Adedokun OJ, Sandborn WJ, Feagan BG, et al. Association between serum concentration of infliximab and efficacy in adult patients with ulcerative colitis. *Gastroenterology* 2014;147:1296–1307.

[51] Reinisch W, Colombel JF, Sandborn WJ, et al. Factors associated with short- and long-term outcomes of therapy for crohn's disease. *Clin Gastroenterol Hepatol* 2015;13:539–547.

[52] Warman A, Straathof JWA, Derijks LJJ. Therapeutic drug monitoring of infliximab in inflammatory bowel disease patients in a teaching hospital setting: results of a prospective cohort study. *Eur J Gastroenterol Hepatol* 2015; 27:242–248.

[53] Arias MT, Vande Casteele N, Vermeire S, et al. A panel to predict long-term outcome of infliximab therapy for patients with ulcerative colitis. *Clin Gastroenterol Hepatol* 2015;13:531–538.

[54] Bortlik M, Duricova D, Malickova K, et al. Infliximab trough levels may predict sustained response to inflix-imab in patients with Crohn's disease. *J Crohns Colitis* 2013;7:736–743.

[55] Singh N, Rosenthal CJ, Melmed GY, et al. Early infliximab trough levels are associated with persistent remission in pediatric patients with inflammatory bowel disease. *Inflamm Bowel Dis* 2014;20:1708–1713.

[56] Roblin X, Marotte H, Rinaudo M, et al. Association between pharmacokinetics of adalimumab and mucosal healing in patients with

inflammatory bowel diseases. *Clin Gastroenterol Hepatol* 2014;12:80–84.

[57] Mazor Y, Almog R, Kopylov U, et al. Adalimumab drug and antibody levels as predictors of clinical and laboratory response in patients with Crohn's disease. *Aliment Pharmacol Ther* 2014;40:620–628.

[58] Ward MG, Kariyawasam VC, Mogan SB, et al. Clinical utility of measuring adalimumab trough levels and antibodies to adalimumab in patients with inflammatory bowel diseases. *J Gastroenterol Hepatol* 2013; 28:100–101.

[59] Steenholdt C, Frederiksen MT, Bendtzen K, et al. Time course and clinical implications of development of antibodies against adalimumab in patients with inflammatory bowel disease. *J Clin Gastroenterol* 2016;50:483–489.

[60] Frederiksen MT, Ainsworth MA, Brynskov J, et al. Antibodies against infliximab (IFX) are associated with de novo development of antibodies to adalimumab (ADL) and therapeutic failure in IFX-to-ADL switchers with inflammatory bowel disease. *Inflamm Bowel Dis* 2014; 20:1714–1721.

[61] Chaparro M, Guerra I, Iborra M, et al. Correlation between adalimumab serum levels and remission after the induction phase in crohn's disease patients. *Gastroenterology* 2015;148:S107–S108.

[62] Vande Casteele N, Feagan B, Vermeire S, et al. Covariates influencing the exposure-response relationship for certolizumab pegol during the induction and maintenances phases in patients with Crohn's disease. *Am J Gastroenterol* 2016;111:S262–S263.

[63] Ungar B, Levy I, Yavne Y, et al. Optimizing anti-TNF-alpha therapy: Serum levels of infliximab and adalimumab are associated with mucosal healing in patients with inflammatory bowel diseases. *Clin Gastroenterol Hepatol* 2016;14(4):550,557.e2.

[64] Adedokun OJ, Sandborn WJ, Feagan BG, et al. Association between serum concentration of infliximab and efficacy in adult patients with ulcerative colitis. *Gastroenterology* 2014;147:1296–1307.

[65] Gonczi L, Vegh Z, Golovics PA et al. Prediction of Short- and Medium-term Efficacy of Biosimilar Infliximab Therapy. Do Trough

Levels and Antidrug Antibody Levels or Clinical and Biochemical Markers Play the More Important Role? *J Crohns Colitis.* 2017 Jun 1;11(6):697-705.

[66] Vande Casteele N, Mould D, Tops S, et al. Initial Adequate Trough Concentrations during Induction Therapy Correlate with Sustained TNF Suppression and Predict Remission with Adalimumab in Anti-TNF Naïve Crohn's Disease Patients. *Journal of Crohn's and Colitis,* 2015, S18–S76.

[67] Yanai H, Lichtenstein L, Assa A, et al. Levels of drug and antidrug antibodies are associated with outcome of interventions after loss of response to infliximab or adalimumab. *Clin Gastroenterol Hepatol* 2015;13:522–530.

[68] Feuerstein JD, Nguyen GC, Kupfer SS et al. American Gastroenterological Association Institute Guideline on Therapeutic Drug Monitoring in Inflammatory Bowel Disease. *Gastroenterology.* 2017 Sep;153(3):827-834.

[69] Dignass A, Van Assche G, Lindsay JO et al. The second European evidence-based Consensus on the diagnosis and management of Crohn's disease: Current management. *J Crohns Colitis* 2010;4:28-62.

[70] D'Haens GR, Panaccione R, Higgins PD et al. The London Position Statement of the World Congress of Gastroenterology on Biological Therapy for IBD with the European Crohn's and Colitis Organization: when to start, when to stop, which drug to choose, and how to predict response? *Am J Gastroenterol* 2011;106:199-212.

[71] Sandborn WJ, Rutgeerts P, Enns R, et al. Adalimumab induction therapy for Crohn disease previously treated with infliximab: a randomized trial. *Ann Intern Med.* 2007;146:829-38.

[72] Ma C, Panaccione R, Heitman SJ, et al. Systematic review: the short-term and long-term efficacy of adalimumab following discontinuation of infliximab. *Aliment Pharmacol Ther.* 2009;30:977-86.

[73] Ben-Horin S, Chowers Y. Review article: loss of response to anti-TNF treatments in Crohn's disease. *Aliment Pharmacol Ther.* 2011;33:987-95.

[74] Sandborn WJ, Abreu MT, D'Haens G et al. Certolizumab pegol in patients with moderate to severe Crohn's disease and secondary failure to infliximab. *Clin Gastroenterol Hepatol* 2010;8:688-695.

[75] Steenholdt C, Brynskov J, Thomsen OØ, et al. Individualised therapy is more cost-effective than dose intensification in patients with Crohn's disease who lose response to anti-TNF treatment: a randomised, controlled trial. *Gut* 2014;63:919–27.

[76] Steenholdt C, Brynskov J, Thomsen OØ, et al. Individualized therapy is a long-term cost-effective method compared to dose intensification in Crohn's disease patients failing infliximab. *Dig Dis Sci* 2015;60:2762–70.

[77] Afif W, Loftus EV Jr, Faubion WA et al. Clinical utility of measuring infliximab and human anti-chimeric antibody concentrations in patients with inflammatory bowel disease. *Am J Gastroenterol* 2010;105:1133–9.

[78] Roblin X, Rinaudo M, Del Tedesco E, et al. Development of an algorithm incorporating pharmacokinetics of adalimumab in inflammatory bowel diseases. *Am J Gastroenterol* 2014;109:1250–6.

[79] R. Khanna, B. D. Sattin, W. Afif et al., Review article: a clinician's guide for therapeutic drug monitoring of infliximab in inflammatory bowel disease. *Aliment Pharmacol Ther* 2013; 38: 447–459.

[80] Ben-Horin S, Waterman M, Kopylov U, et al. Addition of an immunomodulator to infliximab therapy eliminates antidrug antibodies in serum and restores clinical response of patients with inflammatory bowel disease. *Clin Gastroenterol Hepatol: Off Clin Pract J Am Gastroenterol Assoc.* 2013;11(4):444–447.

[81] Steenholdt C, Al-Khalaf M, Brynskov J et al. Clinical implications of variations in anti-infliximab antibody levels in patients with inflammatory bowel disease. *Inflamm Bowel Dis* 2012;18:2209-2217.

[82] Ungar B, Chowers Y, Yavzori M et al. The temporal evolution of antidrug antibodies in patients with inflammatory bowel disease treated with infliximab. *Gut* 2014;63:1258-1264.

[83] Vande Casteele N, Gils A, Singh S et al. Antibody response to infliximab and its impact on pharmacokinetics can be transient. *Am J Gastroenterol* 2013;108:962-971.

[84] Velayos FS, Kahn JG, Sandborn WJ, et al. A test-based strategy is more cost effective than empiric dose escalation for patients with Crohn's disease who lose responsiveness to infliximab. *Clin Gastroenterol Hepatol* 2013;11:654-666.

[85] Papamichael K, Gils A, Rutgeerts P et al. Role for therapeutic drug monitoring during induction therapy with TNF antagonists in IBD: evolution in the definition and management of primary nonresponse. *Inflamm Bowel Dis* 2015;21:182-197.

[86] Yarur AJ, Rubin DT. Therapeutic Drug Monitoring of Anti-tumor Necrosis Factor Agents in Patients with Inflammatory Bowel Diseases. *Inflamm Bowel Dis* 2015;21:1709-1718.

[87] Vande Casteele N, Feagan BG, Gils A et al. Therapeutic drug monitoring in inflammatory bowel disease: current state and future perspectives. *Curr Gastroenterol Rep* 2014;16:378.

[88] Vande Casteele N, Gils A. Pharmacokinetics of anti-TNF monoclonal antibodies in inflammatory bowel disease: Adding value to current practice. *J Clin Pharmacol* 2015;55 Suppl 3:S39-S50.

[89] Baert F, Kondragunta V, Lockton S et al. Antibodies to adalimumab are associated with future inflammation in Crohn's patients receiving maintenance adalimumab therapy: a posthoc analysis of the Karmiris trial. *Gut* 2016 Jul;65(7):1126-31.

[90] Cornillie F, Hanauer SB, Diamond RH et al. Postinduction serum infliximab trough level and decrease of C-reactive protein level are associated with durable sustained response to infliximab: a retrospective analysis of the ACCENT I trial. *Gut* 2014;63:1721-1727.

[91] Vermeire S, Gils A. Value of drug level testing and antibody assays in optimising biological therapy. *Front Gastroenterol.* 2012;4(1):41–3.

[92] Rutgeerts P, Sandborn WJ, Feagan BG et al. Infliximab for induction and maintenance therapy for ulcerative colitis. *N Engl J Med* 2005;353:2462-2476.

[93] Colombel JF, Sandborn WJ, Rutgeerts P et al. Adalimumab for maintenance of clinical response and remission in patients with Crohn's disease: the CHARM trial. *Gastroenterology* 2007;132:52-65.

[94] Cleynen I, Vermeire S. Paradoxical inflammation induced by anti-TNF agents in patients with IBD. *Nat Rev Gastroenterol Hepatol.* 2012;9(9):496–503.

[95] Vaughn BP, Martinez-Vazquez M, Patwardhan VR, et al. Proactive therapeutic concentration monitoring of infliximab may improve outcomes for patients with inflammatory bowel disease: results from a pilot observational study. *Inflamm Bowel Dis* 2014;20:1996–2003.

[96] Papamichael K, Van Stappen T, Vande Casteele N, et al. Infliximab concentration thresholds during induction therapy are associated with short-term mucosal healing in patients with ulcerative colitis. *Clin Gastroenterol Hepatol* 2016 Apr;14(4):543-9.

[97] D'Haens G, Vermeire S, Lambrecht G, et al. Drug-level based dosing versus symptombased dose adaptation in patients with crohn's disease: a prospective, randomized multicenter study (TAILORIX). *Gastroenterology* 2016;150:S143.

[98] Pariente B, Laharie D. Review article: why, when and how to de-escalate therapy in inflammatory bowel diseases. *Aliment Pharmacol Ther* 2014;40:338-353.

[99] Papamichael K, Vermeire S. Withdrawal of anti-tumour necrosis factor alpha therapy in inflammatory bowel disease. *World J Gastroenterol* 2015;21:4773-4778.

[100] Siegel CA, Marden SM, Persing SM, et al. Risk of lymphoma associated with combination anti-tumor necrosis factor and immunomodulator therapy for the treatment of Crohn's disease: a meta-analysis. *Clin Gastroenterol Hepatol* 2009;7:874-881.

[101] Louis E, Mary JY, Vernier-Massouille G, et al. Maintenance of remission among patients with Crohn's disease on antimetabolite therapy after infliximab therapy is stopped. *Gastroenterology.* 2012;142:63–70.e5.

[102] Steenholdt C, Molazahi A, Ainsworth MA, et al. Outcome after discontinuing infliximab in patients with inflammatory bowel disease in clinical remission: An observational Danish single center study. *Scand J Gastroenterol.* 2012;47:518-527.

[103] Papamichael K, Vande Casteele N, Gils A et al. Long-term outcome of patients with Crohn's disease who discontinued infliximab therapy upon clinical remission. *Clin Gastroenterol Hepatol* 2015;13:1103-1110.

[104] Waugh AW, Garg S, Matic K, Gramlich L, Wong C, Sadowski DC, Millan M, Bailey R, Todoruk D, Cherry R, et al. Maintenance of clinical benefit in Crohn's disease patients after discontinuation of infliximab: long-term follow-up of a single centre cohort. *Aliment Pharmacol Ther.* 2010;32:1129–1134.

[105] Molander P, Farkkila M, Salminen K et al. Outcome after discontinuation of TNFalpha-blocking therapy in patients with inflammatory bowel disease in deep remission. *Inflamm Bowel Dis* 2014;20:1021-1028.

[106] Farkas K, Lakatos PL, Nagy F. Predictors of relapse in patients with ulcerative colitis in remission after one-year of infliximab therapy. *Scand J Gastroenterol.* 2013 Dec;48(12):1394-8.

[107] Molnár T, Lakatos PL, Farkas K et al. Predictors of relapse in patients with Crohn's disease in remission after 1 year of biological therapy. *Aliment Pharmacol Ther.* 2013 Jan;37(2):225-33.

[108] Drobne D, Bossuyt P, Breynaert C et al. Withdrawal of immunomodulators after co-treatment does not reduce trough level of infliximab in patients with Crohn's disease. *Clin Gastroenterol Hepatol.* 2015 Mar;13(3):514-521.e4.

[109] Gisbert JP, Marin AC, Chaparro M. Systematic review: factors associated with relapse of inflammatory bowel disease after discontinuation of anti-TNF therapy. *Aliment Pharmacol Ther* 2015;42:391-405.

[110] Ben-Horin S, Chowers Y, Ungar B et al. Undetectable anti-TNF drug levels in patients with long-term remission predict successful drug withdrawal. *Aliment Pharmacol Ther* 2015;42:356-364.

In: Advances in Health and Disease. Volume 4 ISBN: 978-1-53613-345-5
Editor: Lowell T. Duncan

Chapter 4

ATORVASTATIN: PREVENTION AND TREATMENT OF DYSLIPIDEMIA IN CLINICAL AND EXPERIMENTAL MEDICINE

T. A. Korolenko[1], T. P. Johnston[2], M. S. Cherkanova[1], N. V. Goncharova[1], V. A. Vavilin[3,4], A. B. Shintyapina[3], N. P. Bgatova[5] and V. I. Kaledin[4]

[1]Institute of Physiology and Basic Medicine, Novosibirsk, Russia
[2]Division of Pharmaceutical Sciences,
University of Missouri-Kansas City, Kansas City, MO, US
[3]Institute of Molecular Biology and Biophysics, Novosibirsk, Russia
[4]Institute of Cytology and Genetics,
Siberian Branch of Russian Academy of Sciences (SB RAS),
Novosibirsk, Russia
[5]Institute of Clinical and Experimental Lymphology,
Branch of Institute of Cytology and Genetics,
SB RAS, Novosibirsk, Russia

INTRODUCTION

The use of statins is necessary for the prevention and treatment of atherosclerosis, and the criteria for assessing their hypolipidemic effect are clearly defined. Atorvastatin is one of the most commonly prescribed statins in cardiology and other branches of clinical medicine. The pleiotropic effects of statins have not been thoroughly studied until now. In clinical practice, results of a high-sensitivity C-reactive protein (hs-CRP) assay, which reflect the anti-inflammatory effect of various drugs, are commonly analyzed. It appears to be relevant at present to evaluate the effects of statins on changes in new biochemical markers of a nonlipid nature that reflect the progression of atherosclerosis and the involvement of activated macrophages in the pathogenesis.

Atorvastatin treatment of patients with ischemic heart disease and atherosclerosis decreases serum hs-CRP results and serum interleukin 6 and TNF-α concentrations. It was noted that the use of statins decreases both the activity and expression of matrix metalloproteases (MMPs) in atherosclerotic plaques. Although high levels of low-density lipoprotein (LDL)-cholesterol, low levels of HDL-cholesterol, and increased activity of MMPs are common risk factors for ischemic heart disease, it remains unclear how the activities of other possible biomarkers of nonlipid nature (like chitotriosidase, MMPs, and the concentration of cystatin C) change at different stages of the disease and during treatment with atorvastatin. Therefore, it would be worthwhile to evaluate the changes in the activity of chitotriosidase and MMPs and a cystatin C concentration in relation to both lipid indices and changes in hs-CRP results in the serum of patients with atherosclerosis and those who are being treated with statins, especially after myocardial revascularization by a coronary bypass.

It has been shown experimentally that, depending on the severity of experimental hyperlipoproteinemia, oral administration of atorvastatin has a different effect on the overall activity of MMPs in the serum of mice. An increase in the activity of chitotriosidase in the serum of atorvastatin-treated mice is known to be independent of the severity of experimental hyperlipoproteinemia, whereas changes in the activity of MMPs during atorvastatin treatment positively correlate with the severity of experimentally induced hyperlipoproteinemia.

Cardiovascular Pathology: Cysteine Proteases and Their Endogenous Inhibitors

Early diagnosis and reversibility of changes observed during atherosclerosis are important for clinical medicine and to the patients affected by this disease (Johnston et al., 2017a, b). It has been shown that protein degradation by different proteases is partly responsible for cardiovascular dysfunction in various types of heart diseases, including atherosclerosis (Brömme, Wilson, 2011; Korolenko et al., 2012, 2013, 2014). Some evidence has been obtained supporting the hypothesis that the proteolytic activity of cathepsin B reflects the inflammatory component of atherosclerotic pathology and can reflect the antiatherosclerotic therapeutic effects of statins (Lutgens et al., 2007; Kim et al., 2009). The emerging roles of cysteine proteases are related to their potential as drug targets (Turk et al., 2001; Stoka et al., 2005; Kaminskyy, Zhivotovsky, 2012). The first study showed that macrophage-secreted cathepsin B activity in atheroma can be attenuated by photodynamic therapy using a protease-mediated "therapeutic" agent (Shon et al., 2013). Nonetheless, the involvement of different classes of proteases in the onset of early atherosclerosis, neurological disorders, and stroke in humans is still not known (Qin, Shi, 2011; Pislar, Kos, 2014) and neither is the role of these enzymes during effective antiatherosclerotic therapy by hypolipidemic drugs, like statins (Ye et al., 2015). This is one of the many reasons why experimental animal models that can reliably recapitulate the phenotypic signatures or manifestations of human atherosclerosis are so useful for investigating the dynamic processes associated with this disease state.

Lipid accumulation in macrophages was observed in a mouse model of P-407-induced atherosclerosis (Johnston, 2010). Macrophage storage syndrome with lipids and/or P-407 can induce disturbances in lysosomal function of these cells, which may play an important role in the mechanism of atherosclerotic foam cell formation (Lutgens et al., 2007; Qin & Shi, 2011). According to the literature, an increase in cathepsin B activity is detectable *in vivo* and *in vitro* during incubation of hyperlipidemic postprandial serum with monocyte-derived macrophages (Jaffer et al., 2008). Macrophages express several lysosomal cysteine proteases such as cathepsins and legumain (Solberg et al., 2015).

It has been suggested that an inadequate response of activity of lysosomal enzymes owing to lipid overload may contribute to the development of atherosclerotic foam cells. These results also indicate that lipid accumulation blunts autophagic proteolysis via impairment of autophagosomal acidification and cathepsin expression (Inami et al., 2011). Specific functions of lysosomal proteases in endocytic and autophagic pathways have been discussed (Muller et al., 2012). Those authors have summarized the functions of individual endolysosomal proteases in such processes as lipoprotein particle degradation, antigen presentation, and autophagy. Previously it was suggested that the proteases responsible for lysosomal degradation of low-density lipoprotein (LDL) include endolysosomal cathepsins B and D (Svechnikova et al., 1998); although later it was shown that macrophages in atheroma containing abundant cysteine cathepsins K and S contribute to extracellular matrix (ECM) remodeling because of their elastinolytic and collagenolytic activities. Lysosomal damage can occur after uptake of lipoproteins (and cholesterol crystals) by macrophages. The cathepsins are then released into the cytosol where they activate the NLRP3 inflammasome by an unknown mechanism (Muller et al., 2012). Serine carboxypeptidase cathepsin A (substrate: lysosome-associated membrane protein type 2a, LAMP2A) is one protease that had been shown to be crucial for chaperone-mediated autophagy (CMA), aa well as cathepsins D and L are important for macroautophagy (Muller et al., 2012; Repnik et al., 2013).

We have shown that acute lipemia in mice induced by P-407 is followed by increased activities of lysosomal cysteine proteases cathepsin B, cathepsin L, and aspartate protease cathepsin D in the heart tissue of CBA mice (Figure 1), 24 h after P-407 administration, a time point post-dosing at which significant lipemia (cholesterolemia and especially trigliceridemia) develops (Johnston, 2004; Johnston et al., 2017; Korolenko et al., 2016). Increased cathepsin D activity in the heart of mice was also noted later, on the 5th day after acute lipemia (Figure 1), which demonstrates the possibility of further injury of the heart tissue (Korolenko, Johnston, 2015).

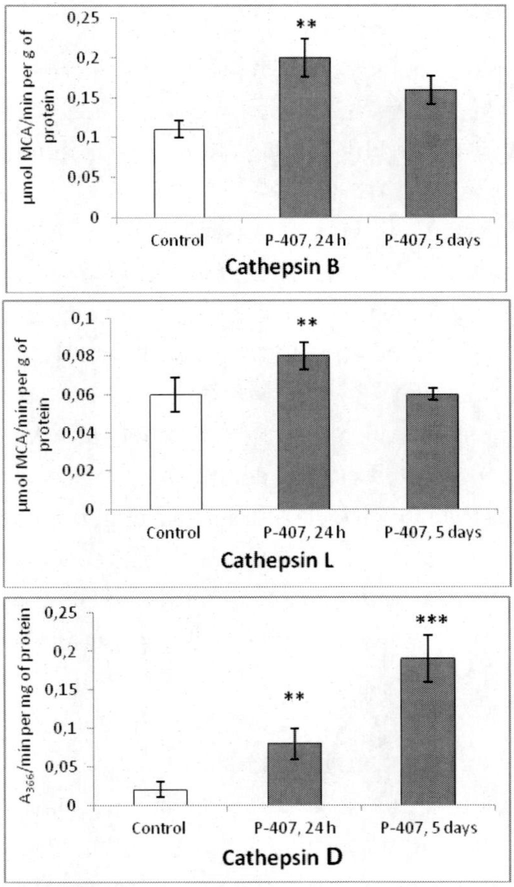

**p < 0.01; ***p < 0.001 vs control.

Figure 1. Cysteine and aspartic protease specific activity in the heart of mice after P-407 (500 mg/kg, single dose, 24 h) administration (M ± m).

Notes: Cathepsin B and cathepsin L specific activity is expressed in µmol MCA/min per g protein, where MCA: 4-methylcoumarylamide.

Cathepsin D specific activity is expressed in A_{366}/min per mg protein.

P-407 is a known general lipase inhibitor (Johnston, 2010). Presumably, lysosomal acid lipase (LAL) would be inhibited as well as in the presence of P-407. *LAL* gene expression was found to decrease *in the liver* of mice during acute lipemia, with significant restoration in mice with lipemia pretreated with atorvastatin or fenofibrate (Shintyapina et al., unpublished data). In the liver, lipid droplets can be delivered to lysosomes via autophagy, where LAL hydrolyzes cholesteryl esters of lipid droplets with formation of free cholesterol mainly for cellular export by the ABCA1 (ATP-binding cassette transporter); this process is specifically induced during macrophage cholesterol loading. A similar process can take place in acute lipemia that is induced by Triton WR 1339, which inhibits acid lipase *in vivo* (Zarzecki et al., 2014).

The level of cystatin C in serum is the most important endogenous inhibitor of cathepsin B (Ge et al., 2012; Korolenko et al., 2011), revealing except inhibition of cysteine proteases various biological effects (Zhu et al., 2015). Human cystatin C belongs to the cystatin family (the extracellular type 2 cystatins, according to the MEROPS classification), which are endogenous low-molecular-weight proteins with a basic function related to inhibition of cysteine proteases and control of proteolysis (Grubb et al., 2010). Cystatin C is the most widely studied cystatin, involved in aging, cell death, degradation of proteins in the ECM, cell differentiation, proliferation and migration of some cell types, synthesis of interleukins and NO (Mathews, Levy, 2016) as well as in antigen processing and presentation (Wallin et al., 2013). Cystatin C is a low-molecular-weight non-lipid biomarker and risk factor of acute cardiovascular events in patients with cardiovascular pathology. Our recent data revealed a direct correlation between the levels of cystatin C, urea, creatinine, and NT-proBNP (a precursor of brain natriuretic peptide) known as the risk factors of acute cardiovascular complications and predictors of restenosis after coronary stenting; these findings point to the utility of cystatin C as a marker of not only renal failure but also cardiovascular pathology (Gevorgyan et al., 2017). In comparison with other biomarkers, cystatin C can be regarded as a potential predictor of cardiovascular complications in patients with atherosclerosis and coronary heart diseases, although it is not as predictive as CRP-hs or NT-proBNP. The function of cystatin C is related to the protection of the human body from the damaging action of extracellular cysteine proteases, which are inactivated after binding to endogenous inhibitors, and the most potent mechanism is exemplified by the cathepsin B/cystatin C ratio (Gevorgyan et al., 2017).

Poloxamer 407-Induced and Triton WR 1339-Induced Experimental Models of Hyperlipidemia and Atherosclerosis

P-407 is a known general lipase inhibitor and inhibitor of LAL (Johnston, 2010). Thus, it has been widely used to reproduce acute lipemia and atherosclerosis at different stages of development in rodents in experimental studies development, since inhibition of key lipases involved with lipid metabolism, such as hepatic lipase, lipoprotein lipase, and endothelial lipase, cause disturbances to lipid and lipoprotein levels (Johnston, 2010). The protective hypolipidemic effect of atorvastatin pretreatment has been shown in our study in this model of acute murine lipemia using a P-407 dose of 500 mg/kg (Figure 2). Atorvastatin decreased serum concentrations of total cholesterol, non-HDL cholesterol, and TGs but not to the levels in untreated mice with a tendency for elevation of serum HDL-cholesterol (Figure 2).

A similar protective effect of atorvastatin pretreatment (at the dose of 75 mg/kg, twice) was demonstrated in another model of acute lipemia induced by single administration of the same dose of another lysosomotropic agent, Triton WR 1339 (Figure 3).

There was also an increased level of both total serum cholesterol and especially TGs, whereas atorvastatin significantly decreased these parameters, but not to the levels of control mice (Figure 3). Thus, in two murine models of acute lipemia there were similarities in characteristics of lipemia and in the mechanism of hypolipidemic effects of both P-407 and Triton WR 1339 lipemia (Loginova et al., 2013).

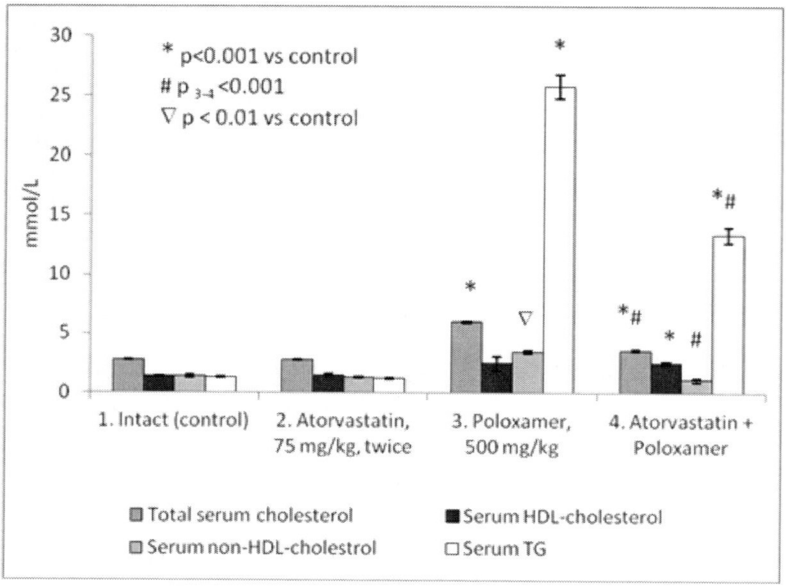

Figure 2. The influence of atorvastatin on P-407–induced lipemia in CBA mice (mmol/L).

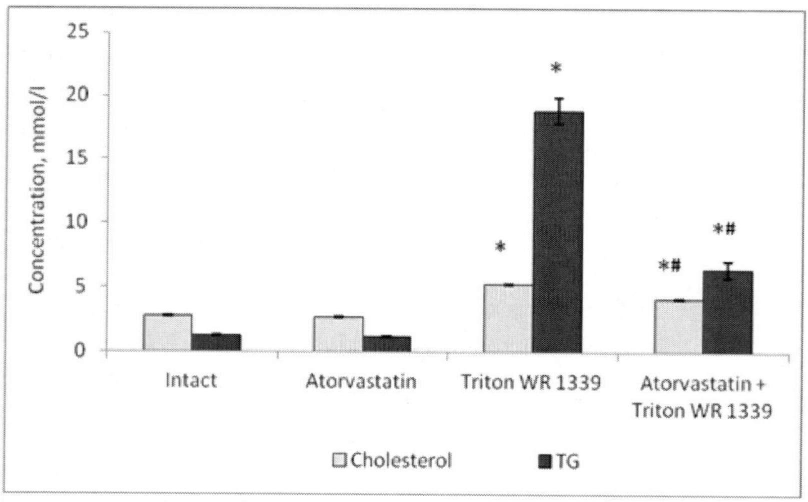

Notes: *p < 0.001 vs control; #p < 0.001 atorvastatin + Triton WR 1339 vs Triton WR 1339.

Figure 3. The influence of atorvastatin pretreatment on Triton WR 1339–induced lipemia in CBA mice (mmol/L).

PLEIOTROPIC EFFECTS OF STATINS

The use of statins is necessary for the treatment and prevention of atherosclerosis; criteria for assessing their hypolipidemic effect are clearly defined (Collins et al., 2016). It is known that statin treatment in addition to lipid-lowering exerts pleiotropic effects (Scheme). Moreover, there is some specificity of biological effects of different statins (for example, hypolipidemic activity and other effects of atorvastatin vs pravastatin and other statins) (Qian et al., 2015; Melendez et al., 2017). It was reported that in high doses, atorvastatin's positive effect is superior to that of moderate-dose simvastatin in preventing peripheral arterial disease (Stoekenbroek et al., 2015). In general, in patients with ischemic heart disease treated with statins, there is a decrease in serum hs-CRP readings (Jaffer et al., 2008; Cherkanova et al., 2012) and in interleukin 6 and TNF-α levels (Han et al., 2017), indicating their anti-inflammatory effect. In an experiment reproducing acute lipemia in mice, similar results were obtained (Goncharova et al., 2016), revealing lipid-lowering and some anti-inflammatory activity of atorvastatin (Korolenko et al., 2012; 2016 a,b).

The literature data on the relation between changes in different types of MMPs and serum lipids during treatment with statins have been discussed (Wu et al., 2005; Korolenko, Johnston, 2015). It seems relevant to study the effect of statins on changes in new nonlipid biochemical markers that reflect the progression of atherosclerosis and the involvement of activated macrophages in the pathogenesis. Depending on the severity of experimental hyperlipidemia, oral administration of atorvastatin (at the same dose) exerts a different effect on the total serum activity of MMP in mice: increases MMP activity after “moderate” induction by P-407, 500 mg/kg, and decreases during “significant” acute lipemia induced by P-407 (1000 mg/kg). In mice with “moderate” experimental lipemia, atorvastatin manifests a hypolipidemic effect, whereas in mice with “significant” lipemia, the protective hypolipidemic effect of atorvastatin has not been registered (Korolenko et al., 2009; Cherkanova et al., 2012). The total serum MMP activity that we measured in our study was determined by an enzymatic assay that provided information on several MMP types, including mostly gelatinases (MMP-2 and MMP-9) and matrilysin (MMP-7). According to a more recent proteome analysis, this assay may cross-react with other types of MMPs, like stromelysins (MMP-3, -10, -11), all of which participate in plaque instability (Dufour, Overall, 2013). The advantage of the MMP activity assay that we used is that it identifies only the active forms of the enzymes, not enzymatically inactive proenzymes or MMP complexes with either endogenous TIMPs or α_2-macroglobulin.

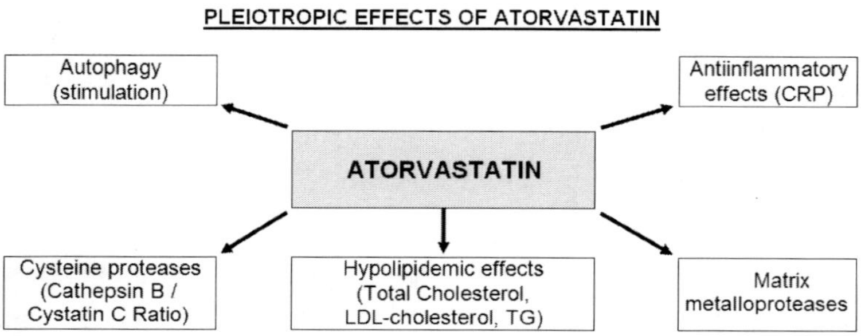

Scheme

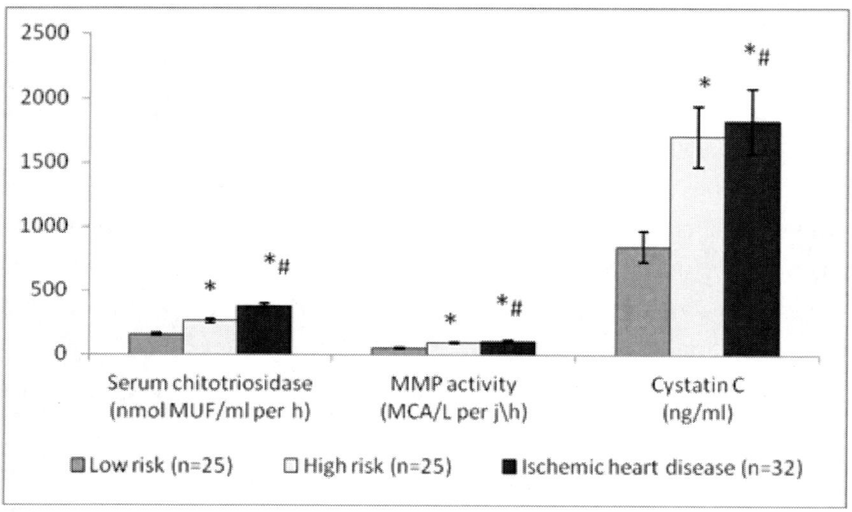

Notes: *p < 0.001 vs the group of low risk; #p < 0.05 vs the group of high risk.

Figure 4. Serum chitotriosidase and MMP activities and cystatin C concentration in patients at different risks of ischemic heart disease.

In patients with ischemic heart diseases, there is evidence of an increase in serum chitotriosidase and MMP activity, which correlate with the risk of ischemic heart disease (Figure 4).

Atorvastatin: Induction of Autophagy

Autophagy (self-eating) is an important cellular process closely related to functioning of the endolysosomal system, including endocytosis and exocytosis (Mizushima et al., 2008). Autophagy plays an important role in cellular homeostasis, essential for heart and vessel homeostasis and function; however, defective or excessive autophagic activity seems to contribute to major cardiovascular disorders including atherosclerosis (Mialet-Perez, Vindis, 2017). Defects in autophagy linked to a wide range of diseases have given rise to the hypothesis that autophagy inducers can prevent or treat certain clinical conditions related to decreased autophagy (Galluzzi et al., 2017; Levine et al., 2017). Atorvastatin has been demonstrated to stimulate autophagy in a nonischemic myocardium while partly inhibiting autophagy in an ischemic myocardium (Yang et al., 2010; Sabe et al., 2014). Atorvastatin may effectively activate autophagy via the AMPK–mTOR (AMP activated protein kinase–mammalian target of rapamycin) pathway to enhance mesenchymal stem cell survival during hypoxia and/or serum deprivation in some cell lines (Wang et al., 2015; Zhang et al., 2012) and in spontaneously hypertensive rats (Wang et al., 2015).

Induction of autophagy by atorvastatin was detected in mesenchymal stem cells during hypoxia and serum deprivation (Li N. et al, 2014). At the same time, inhibition of autophagy can potentiate atorvastatin-induced apoptotic cell death in human bladder cancer cells *in vitro* (Kang et al., 2014; King et al., 2016).

Autophagy is important as a novel therapeutic target with a wide range of beneficial effects on human diseases, including cardiovascular and neurodegenerative pathology and cancer (Maxfield, 2014; Korolenko et al.,

2017). Novel pharmacological modulators of autophagy, including statins, have been presented (Hale et al., 2013; Ha, Kim, 2016). Atorvastatin has been shown to stimulate autophagy in a nonischemic myocardium while partly inhibiting autophagy in an ischemic myocardium (Yang et al., 2010; Sabe et al., 2014; Liang et al., 2017). According to recent data, atorvastatin can effectively activate autophagy via the AMPK–mTOR pathway thereby enhancing mesenchymal stem cell survival during hypoxia and/or serum deprivation in some cell lines (Zhang et al., 2012) and in spontaneously hypertensive rats (Wang et al., 2015). AMPK-mediated cardioprotection by atorvastatin was suggested to be related to a reduction in apoptosis and activation of autophagy in infarcted rat hearts (Li et al., 2016).

Atorvastatin is believed to have anticancer effects related to autophagy (Chen., Klionsky, 2011; Feng, et al., 2015). Statins have been reported to offer cancer-preventive benefits including a reduction in the risk of prostate cancer (Parikh et al., 2010; He et al., 2015). Atorvastatin has been demonstrated to act as an inducer of autophagy in androgen receptor–negative prostate cancer PC3 cells through inhibition of geranylgeranyl biosynthesis. Atorvastatin treatment elevated LC-II in PC3 cells, and this process is dependent on inhibition of the biosynthesis of geranylgeranyl. It was proposed that the inhibition of geranylgeranyl biosynthesis by atorvastatin activates transcription of LC3, which results in upregulation of LC3-II and activation of autophagy (Toepfer et al., 2011). In human A172 glioma, atorvastatin was shown to promote cytotoxicity and reduce migration and proliferation of tumor cells (Oliveira et al., 2017).

Atorvastatin protects vascular smooth muscle cells from TGF-β1–stimulated calcification by inducing autophagy via suppression of the β-catenin pathway (Liu et al., 2014). Atorvastatin improves an inflammatory response in atherosclerosis by upregulating GARP (a newly identified biological membrane molecule on activated regulatory T cells [Tregs], in conjunction with the release of TGF-β in an atherosclerotic plaque); possibly, by this mechanism, atorvastatin can delay the progression of atherosclerosis and improve stability of atherosclerotic plaques (Zhao et al., 2015). Moreover, antioxidant and antiplatelet effects of atorvastatin via NOX2 inhibition were shown in a clinical study (Violi et al., 2014)

Autophagy induced by atorvastatin can promote recovery neurological function (Gao et al., 2016).

ATORVASTATIN VS COMBINED EFFECTS OF ATORVASTATIN AND FENOFIBRATE IN EXPERIMENTAL LIPEMIA

In several clinical studies, it has been revealed that combination therapy (atorvastatin and fenofibrate) is safe and has beneficial additive effects on endothelial function in patients with combined hyperlipidemia (Koh et al., 2005; Davidson et al., 2009; 2012) or type 2 diabetes mellitus (Costet et al., 2010; Lella, Indira, 2013). A comparison of atorvastatin and fenofibrate in terms of attainment of lipid targets and biomarkers of endothelial damage in patients with familial combined hyperlipidemia revealed that atorvastatin and fenofibrate significantly improve the lipid profile (Harivenkatesh et al., 2014) and cause a comparable decrease in plasma oxysterols, with the normalization of 7-ketocholesterol and a significant reduction in 7β-hydroxycholesterol concentration; both atorvastatin and fenofibrate showed comparable efficacy in decreasing oxysterol levels (Arco et al., 2007). Nevertheless, the dose-dependent effect of both atorvastatin and fenofibrate and their combinations was not clear. In addition, it was found that a combination of atorvastatin and fenofibrate increases apolipoprotein AV levels (implicated in TG metabolism) and downregulates TGs by upregulating peroxisome proliferator-activated receptor α. (Huang et al., 2009). Downregulation of the apolipoprotein AV gene results in an increase of plasma TG levels in male Sprague-Dawley rats, whereas its overexpression downregulates TGs (Huang et al., 2009).

In an experiment on New Zealand white rabbits with exogenous hypercholesterolemia, an atorvastatin and fenofibrate combination induced predominance of the large HDL subclasses and increased apo AI fractional catabolic rates (Flores-Castillo et al., 2015).

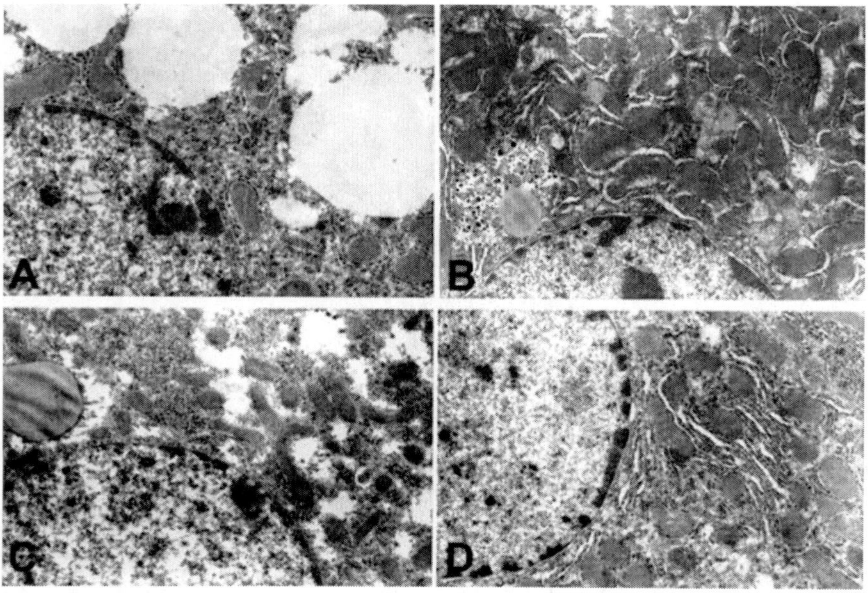

Figure 5. Ultrastructural organization of hepatocytes in mice with P-407–induced acute lipemia pretreated with atorvastatin or/and fenofibrate (Tricor). Magnification 6000×. (A). An increased amount of lipid inclusions of various sizes (from small to very large) in the cytoplasm of a hepatocyte from mice with acute lipemia (P-407, 250 mg/kg, 24 h). (B). Pretreatment with *atorvastatin* significantly decreased lipid content of hepatocytes relative to acute lipemia (P-407, 250 mg/kg, 24 h). (C). The liver of mice with preliminary administration of *fenofibrate* in acute lipemia. In hepatocytes, several lipid inclusions were detected; a decrease in the glycogen content of cells was observed. (D). Hepatocytes during combined administration of atorvastatin and fenofibrate in acute lipemia. There are no lipid droplets in the cytoplasm.

The efficacy of 4 drug regimens (fibrate, ezetimibe, low-dose atorvastatin, and high-dose atorvastatin) for the management of the dyslipidemia of metabolic syndrome in a C57BL6 mouse model has been studied (Paraskevas et al., 2011). The aim of pharmacotherapy was to correct or normalize blood pressure, total cholesterol, LDL-cholesterol (LDL-C), HDL-C, TG, and glucose values. It was concluded that high-dose atorvastatin treatment may be the optimal therapeutic option for the dyslipidemia associated with metabolic syndrome. The effect and safety of an approved combination therapy with simvastatin and fenofibrate are described in a review by Tarantino et al., (2017) with special attention to the toxicity of this combination.

According to our electron microscopic study, atorvastatin or/and fenofibrate (Tricor) pretreatment improves hepatocytic morphology as compared to untreated mice with acute lipemia (received only P-407, 250 mg/kg, 24 h after); however, the most effective was administration of a combination of atorvastatin + fenofibrate resulting in a significant improvement in murine hepatocyte structure and a significantly reduced number of lipid droplets in the cytoplasm (Figure 5).

CONCLUSION

Atorvastatin belongs to the statin class of HMG-Co reductase inhibitors which exert not only a significant hypolipidemic, but also several pleiotropic effects. The new effects of atorvastatin include antiinflammatory effects, antitumor activity, and the stimulation of autophagy. These effects open new possibilities for further study of atorvastatin and its therapeutic clinical applications in different branches of medicine.

ACKNOWLEDGMENTS

The study was partially supported by Russian Foundation for Basic Research (Russia) grant 16-04-01423/17

REFERENCES

Arca, M; Montali, A; Pigna, G; Antonini, R; Antonini, TM; Luigi, P; Fraioli, A; Mastrantoni, M; Maddaloni, M; Letizia, C. Comparison of atorvastatin versus fenofibrate in reaching lipid targets and influencing biomarkers of endothelial damage in patients with familial combined hyperlipidemia. *Metabolism,* 2007, 56(11), 1534-1541.

Brömme, D; Wilson, S. Role of cysteine cathepsins in extracellular proteolysis. Extracellular Matrix Degradation. *Biology of Extracellular Matrix*, 2011, 2, 23–51.

Chen, Y; Klionsky, DJ. The regulation of autophagy - unanswered questions. *J. Cell Sci,* 2011, 124(Pt 2): 161-170.

Cherkanova, MS; Korolenko, TA; Bravve, Iiu; Gerasimova, TP. [Effect of statins on activity of matrix metalloproteases and serum concentration of cystatin C in patients with various risk of development of ischemic heart disease and in patients after coronary artery bypass surgery]. *Kardiologi*ia, 2012, 52(2):23-28.

Collins, R; Reith, C; Emberson, J; Armitage, J; Baigent, C; Blackwell, L; Blumenthal, R; Danesh, J; Smith, GD, DeMets, D; Evans, S; Law, M; MacMahon, S; Martin, S; Neal, B; Poulter, N; Preiss, D; Ridker, P; Roberts, I; Rodgers, A; Sandercock, P; Schulz, K; Sever, P; Simes, J; Smeeth, L; Wald, N; Yusuf, S; Peto, R. Interpretation of the evidence for the efficacy and safety of statin therapy. *Lancet.* 2016, 388(10059), 2532-2561. doi: 10.1016/S0140-6736(16)31357-5.

Costet, P; Hoffmann, MM; Cariou, B; Guyomarc'h Delasalle, B; Konrad, T; Winkler, K. Plasma PCSK9 is increased by fenofibrate and atorvastatin in a non-additive fashion in diabetic patients. *Atherosclerosis*. 2010, 212(1), 246-251. doi: 10.1016/j.atherosclerosis.2010.05.027.

Davidson, MH; Rooney, MW; Drucker, J; Eugene Griffin, H; Oosman, S; Beckert, M; LCP-AtorFen Investigators. Efficacy and tolerability of atorvastatin/fenofibrate fixed-dose combination tablet compared with atorvastatin and fenofibrate monotherapies in patients with dyslipidemia: a 12-week, multicenter, double-blind, randomized, parallel-group study. *Clin. Ther.* 2009, 31(12), 2824-2838. doi: 10.1016/j.clinthera.2009.12.007.

Davidson, M; Rosenson, RS; Maki, KC; Nicholls, SJ; Ballantyne, CM; Setze, C; Carlson, DM; Stolzenbach, J. Study design, rationale, and baseline characteristics: evaluation of fenofibric acid on carotid intima-media thickness in patients with type IIb dyslipidemia with residual risk in addition to atorvastatin therapy (FIRST) trial. *Cardiovasc. Drugs Ther.*, 2012, 26(4), 349-358. doi: 10.1007/s10557-012-6395-z.

Dufour, A; Overall, CM. Missing the target: matrix metalloproteinase antitargets in inflammation and cancer. *Trends Pharmacol. Sci.*, 2013, 34(4), 233-242. doi: 10.1016/j.tips.2013.02.004.

Flores-Castillo, C; Zamora-Pérez, JÁ; Carreón-Torres, E; Arzola-Paniagua, A; Aguilar-Salinas, C; López-Olmos, V; Fragoso, JM; Luna-Luna, M; Rodríguez-Pérez, JM; Franco, M; Vargas-Alarcón, G; Pérez-Méndez, Ó. Atorvastatin and fenofibrate combination induces the predominance of the large HDL subclasses and increased apo AI fractional catabolic rates in New Zealand white rabbits with exogenous hypercholesterolemia. *Fundam. Clin. Pharmacol.,* 2015, 29(4):362-370. doi: 10.1111/fcp.12125.

Feng, Y; Yao, Z; Klionsky, DJ. How to control self-digestion: transcriptional, post-transcriptional, and post-translational regulation of autophagy. *Trends Cell Biol.,* 2015, 25(6): 354-363. doi: 10.1016/j.tcb.2015.02.002.

Galluzzi, L; Bravo-San Pedro, JM; Levine, B; Green, DR; Kroemer, G. Pharmacological modulation of autophagy: therapeutic potential and persisting obstacles. *Nat. Rev. Drug Discov*., 2017, 16(7):487-511. doi: 10.1038/nrd.2017.22.

Gao, S; Zhang, ZM; Shen, ZL; Gao, K; Chang, L; Guo, Y; Li, Z; Wang, W; Wang, AM. Atorvastatin activates autophagy and promotes neurological function recovery after spinal cord injury. *Neural Regen Res.,* 2016, 11(6): 977-982. doi: 10.4103/1673-5374.184498.

Ge, CJ; Lü, SZ; Feng, LX; Huo, Y; Song, XT; Chen, X; Meng, K; Yuan, F. Combined effect of atorvastatin and probucol on plasma cystatin C levels and severity of coronary lesion in patients with borderline coronary lesion. *Chin. Med. J.* (Engl), 2012, 125(14), 2472-2476.

Gevorgyan, MM; Voronina, NP; Goncharova, NV; Kozaruk, TV; Russkikh, GS; Bogdanova, LA; Korolenko, TA. Cystatin C as a Marker of Progressing Cardiovascular Events during Coronary Heart Disease. *Bull. Exp. Biol. Med.,* 2017, 162(4):421-424. doi: 10.1007/s10517-017-3630-4

Goncharova, NV; Khrapova, MV; Pupyshev, AB; Korolenko, ET; Nešéáková, Z; Korolenko, TA. Hypolipidemic Effect of Mannan in

Mice with Acute Lipemia Induced by Poloxamer 407. *Bull. Exp. Biol. Med.*, 2016, 162(1):18-22.

Grubb, A; Blirup-Jensen, S; Lindström, V; Schmidt, C; Althaus, H; Zegers, I; IFCC Working Group on Standardisation of Cystatin C (WG-SCC). First certified reference material for cystatin C in human serum ERM-DA471/IFCC. Clin. *Chem. Lab. Med.,* 2010, 48(11):1619-1621.

Ha, J; Kim, J. Novel pharmacological modulators of autophagy: an updated patent review (2012-2015). *Expert Opin. Ther. Pat.,* 2016, 26(11): 1273-1289.

Hale, AN; Ledbetter, DJ; Gawriluk, TR; Rucker, EB 3rd. Autophagy: regulation and role in development. *Autophagy,* 2013, 9 (7), 951-972. doi: 10.4161/auto.24273.

Han, F; Xiao, QQ; Peng, S; Che, XY; Jiang, LS; Shao, Q; He, B. Atorvastatin ameliorates LPS-induced inflammatory response by autophagy via AKT/mTOR signaling pathway. *J. Cell Biochem.*, 2017, 119(2), 1604-1615. doi: 10.1002/jcb.26320.

Harivenkatesh, N; David, DC; Haribalaji, N; Sudhakar, MK. Efficacy and safety of alternate day therapy with atorvastatin and fenofibrate combination in mixed dyslipidemia: a randomized controlled trial. *J. Cardiovasc. Pharmacol. Ther.*, 2014, 19(3), 296-303. doi: 10.1177/1074248413518968

He, Z; Yuan, J; Qi, P; Zhang, L; Wang, Z. Atorvastatin induces autophagic cell death in prostate cancer cells *in vitro*. *Mol. Med. Rep.*, 2015, 11(6), 4403-4408. doi: 10.3892/mmr.2015.3334.

Huang, XS; Zhao, SP; Bai, L; Hu, M; Zhao, W; Zhang, Q. Atorvastatin and fenofibrate increase apolipoprotein AV and decrease triglycerides by up-regulating peroxisome proliferator-activated receptor-alpha. *Br. J. Pharmacol.,* 2009, 158(3), 706-712. doi: 10.1111/j.1476-5381. 2009.00350.x.

Inami, Y; Yamashina, S; Izumi, K; Ueno, T; Tanida, I; Ikejima, K; Watanabe, S. Hepatic steatosis inhibits autophagic proteolysis via impairment of autophagosomal acidifi cation and cathepsin expression. *Biochem. Biophys. Res. Commun,* 2011, 412: 618–625.

Jaffer, FA; Vinegoni, C; John, MC; Aikawa, E; Gold, HK; Finn, AV; Ntziachristos, V; Libby, P; Weissleder, R. Real-time catheter molecular sensing of inflammation in proteolytically active atherosclerosis. *Circulation,* 2008, 118: 1802–1809.

Johnston, TP. The P-407-induced murine models of dose-controlled hyperlipidemia and atherosclerosis. *J. Cardiovasc. Pharmacol.,* 2004, 43: 595–606.

Johnston, TP; Palmer WK. Mechanism of poloxamer 407-induced hypertriglyceridemia in the rat. *Biochem. Pharmacol.* 1993, 46(6), 1037-1042.

Johnston, TP; Korolenko, TA; Sahebkar, A. The P-407-Induced Mouse Model of Dose-Controlled Hyperlipidemia and Atherosclerosis: Twenty-five Years Later. *J. Cardiovasc. Pharmacol.*, 2017, 70(5), 339-352. doi: 10.1097/FJC.0000000000000522.

Johnston, TP; Korolenko, TA; Pirro, M; Sahebkar, A. Preventing cardiovascular heart disease: Promising nutraceutical and non-nutraceutical treatments for cholesterol management. *Pharmacol. Res.,* 2017a, 120, 219-225. doi: 10.1016/j.phrs.2017.04.008.

Johnston, TP; Korolenko, TA; Bgatova, NP. (2017b). Statins and Yeast Polysaccharides in the Treatment of Hyperlipidemia and Liver Steatosis, Role of Autophagy. In: Editors: Leon V. Berhardt. P., *Advances in Medicine and Biology.* Hauppauge: Nova Science Publishers, vol. 110, pp. 31-60.

Kang, M; Jeong, CW; Ku, JH; Kwak, C; Kim, HH. Inhibition of autophagy potentiates atorvastatin-induced apoptotic cell death in human bladder cancer cells *in vitro. Int. J. Mol. Sci.,* 2014,15(5), 8106-8121. doi: 10.3390/ijms15058106.

Kaminskyy, V; Zhivotovsky, B. Proteases in autophagy. *Biochim Biophys Acta,* 2012, 1824(1): 44-50.

Kim, DE; Kim, JY; Schellingerhout, D; Shon, SM; Jeong, SW; Kim, EJ; Kim, WK. Molecular imaging of cathepsin B proteolytic enzyme activity reflects the inflammatory component of atherosclerotic pathology and can quantitatively demonstrate the antiatherosclerotic therapeutic eff ects of atorvastatin and glucosamine. *Mol. Imaging,* 2009, 8: 291–301.

King, MA; Ganley, IG; Flemington, V. Inhibition of cholesterol metabolism underlies synergy between mTOR pathway inhibition and chloroquine in bladder cancer cells. *Oncogene,* 2016, 35(34), 4518-4528. doi: 10.1038/onc.2015.511.

Koh, KK; Quon, MJ; Han, SH; Chung, WJ; Ahn, JY; Seo, YH; Choi, IS; Shin, EK. Additive beneficial effects of fenofibrate combined with atorvastatin in the treatment of combined hyperlipidemia. *J. Am. Coll. Cardiol.,* 2005, 45(10), 1649-1653.

Korolenko, TA; Johnston, TP. Aspartate protease cathepsin D in liver and heart Injury. In: E. H. Bennington Ed., *Horizons of World Cardiovascular Research,* 2015, Vol. 8, pp. 33-55.

Korolenko, TA; Cherkanova, MS; Korolenko, EC. Effect of atorvastatin on activities of matrix metalloproteinases and chitotriosidase in male and female mice with experimental hyperlipidemia. *Bull. Exp. Biol. Med.*, 2009, 148(3), 369-373.

Korolenko, TA; Cherkanova, MS; Gashenko, EA; Johnston, TP; Bravve, IY. Cystatin C, atherosclerosis and lipid-lowering therapy by statins. In: Eds. J. B. Cohen, L. P. Rysek. *Cystatins: protease inhibitors, biomarkers and immunomodulators,* N,Y., 2011. P. 187-204.

Korolenko, TA; Tuzikov, FV; Cherkanova, MS; Johnston, TP; Tuzikova, NA; Loginova, VM; Filjushina, EE; Kaledin, VI. Influence of atorvastatin and carboxymethylated glucan on the serum lipoprotein profile and MMP activity of mice with lipemia induced by poloxamer 407. *Can. J. Physiol. Pharmacol.*, 2012, 90(2), 141-153. doi: 10.1139/y11-118.

Korolenko TA; Johnston, TP; Dubrovina, NI; Kisarova, YA; Zhanaeva, SY; Cherkanova, MS; Filjushina, EE; Alexeenko, TV; Machova, E; Zhukova, NA. Effect of poloxamer 407 administration on the serum lipids profile, anxiety level and protease activity in the heart and liver of mice. *Interdiscip. Toxicol.,* 2013, 6(1), 18-25. doi: 10.2478/intox-2013-0004.

Korolenko, T; Cherkanova, M; Gerasimova, T; Korolenko, Ts. Matrix metalloproteases, chitotriosidase and cystatin C in long-term study in patients after cardiosurgery In: Kimchi E, Editor. *New Insights into Mechanisms and Management of Heart Disease*. Vancouver, 2014, Monduzzi Editore, International Proceedings Division, 57-86.

Korolenko, TA; Johnston, TP. (2015). Aspartate protease cathepsin D in liver and heart Injury. In: E. H. Bennington Ed., *Horizons of World Cardiovascular Research,* Vol. 8, Nova Science Publ. Pp. 33-55.

Korolenko, TA; Johnston,TP; Tuzikov, FV; Tuzikova, NA; Pupyshev, AB; Spiridonov, VK; Goncharova, NV; Maiborodin, IV; Zhukova, NA. Early-stage atherosclerosis in poloxamer 407-induced hyperlipidemic mice: pathological features and changes in the lipid composition of serum lipoprotein fractions and subfractions. *Lipids in Health and Disease,* 2016a; 15:16. doi: 10.1186/s12944-016-0186-7.

Korolenko, TA; Johnston, TP; Lykov, AP; Shintyapina, AB; Khrapova, MV; Goncharova, NV; Korolenko, E; Bgatova, NP; Machova, E; Nescakova, Z; Sakhno, LV. A comparative study of the hypolipidaemic effects of a new polysaccharide, mannan *Candida albicans* serotype A, and atorvastatin in mice with poloxamer 407-induced hyperlipidaemia. *J. Pharm. Pharmacol.*, 2016b, 68(12), 1516-1526. doi: 10.1111/jphp.12633.

Korolenko, TA; Pupyshev, AB; Pospelova, TI; Gritsyk, OB; Panov, AV; Vavilin, VA; Shintyapina, AB; Tikhonova, MA. Autophagy and neurodegeneration. In: Simon A., Editor. *Neurodegenerative Disease. Overview, Perspectives and Emerging Treatments*. New York, Nova Science Publishers, 2017, 1-33.

Lella, M; Indira, K. A comparative study of efficacy of atorvastatin alone and its combination with fenofibrate on lipid profile in type 2 diabetes mellitus patients with hyperlipidemia. *J. Adv. Pharm. Technol. Res.,* 2013, 4(3), 166-170. doi: 10.4103/2231-4040.116778.

Levine, B; Packer, M; Codogno, P. Development of autophagy inducers in clinical medicine. *The Journal of Clinical Investigation*, 2017, Dec. 8. https://doi.org/10.1172/JCI73938.

Li, N; Zhang, Q; Qian, H; Jin, C; Yang, Y; Gao, R. Atorvastatin induces autophagy of mesenchymal stem cells under hypoxia and serum deprivation conditions by activating the mitogen-activated protein kinase/extracellular signal-regulated kinase pathway. *Chin. Med. J.* (Engl), 2014, 127(6), 1046-1051.

Li, Q; Dong, QT; Yang, YJ; Tian, XQ; Jin, C; Huang, PS; Jiang, LP; Chen, GH. AMPK-mediated cardioprotection of atorvastatin relates to the reduction of apoptosis and activation of autophagy in infarcted rat hearts. *Am. J. Transl. Res.,* 2016, 8(10), 4160-4171. eCollection 2016.

Liang, J; Yin, K; Cao, X; Han, Z; Huang, Q; Zhang, L; Ma, W; Ding, F; Bi, C; Feng, D; Pan, Z; Liu, Y. Attenuation of Low Ambient Temperature-Induced Myocardial Hypertrophy by Atorvastatin via Promoting Bcl-2 Expression. *Cell Physiol. Biochem.*, 2017, 41(1), 286-295. doi: 10.1159/000456111.

Liu, D; Cui, W; Liu, B; Hu, H; Liu, J; Xie, R; Yang, X; Gu, G; Zhang, J; Zheng, H. Atorvastatin protects vascular smooth muscle cells from TGF-β1-stimulated calcification by inducing autophagy via suppression of the β-catenin pathway. *Cell Physiol. Biochem.*, 2014, 33(1), 129-141. doi: 10.1159/000356656.

Loginova, VM; Tuzikov, FV; Tuzikova, NA; Korolenko, TA. Comparative characteristics of lipemia models induced by injections of Triton WR-1339 and poloxamer 407 in mice. *Bull. Exp. Biol. Med.*, 2013, 155(2), 284-287.

Lutgens, SP; Cleutjens, KB; Daemen, MJ; Heeneman, S. Cathepsin cysteine proteases in cardiovascular disease. *FASEB J.,* 2007, 21, 3029–3041.

Mathews, PM; Levy, E. Cystatin C in aging and in Alzheimer's disease. *Ageing Res. Rev.* 2016, 32, 38-50. doi: 10.1016/j.arr.2016.06.003.

Maxfield, FR. Role of endosomes and lysosomes in human disease. *Cold Spring Harb. Perspect. Biol.* 2014, 6(5): a016931. doi: 10.1101/cshperspect.a016931.

Melendez, QM; Wooten, CJ; Lopez, D. Atorvastatin and lovastatin, but not pravastatin, increased cellular complex formation between PCSK9 and the LDL receptor in human hepatocyte-like C3A cells. *Biochem Biophys Res Commun.*, 2017, 492(1), 103-108. doi: 10.1016/j.bbrc.2017.08.026.

Mialet-Perez, J; Vindis, C. Autophagy in health and disease: focus on the cardiovascular system. *Essays Biochem.*, 2017, 61(6),721-732. doi: 10.1042/EBC20170022.

Mizushima, N; Levine, B; Cuervo, AM; Klionsky, DJ. Autophagy fights disease through cellular self-digestion. *Nature,* 2008, 451(7182), 1069-1075. doi: 10.1038/nature06639. Review.

Muller, S; Dennemarker, J; Reinheckel, T. Specific functions of lysosomal proteases in endocytic and autophagic pathways. *BBA,* 2012, 1824(1), 34–43.

Oliveira, KA; Dal-Cim, T; Lopes, FG; Ludka, FK; Nedel, CB; Tasca, CI. Atorvastatin Promotes Cytotoxicity and Reduces Migration and Proliferation of Human A172 Glioma Cells. *Mol. Neurobiol.,* 2017 Feb 8. doi: 10.1007/s12035-017-0423-8.

Paraskevas, KI; Pantopoulou, A; Vlachos, IS; Agrogiannis, G; Iliopoulos, DG; Karatzas, G; Tzivras, D; Mikhailidis, DP; Perrea, DN. Comparison of fibrate, ezetimibe, low- and high-dose statin therapy for the dyslipidemia of the metabolic syndrome in a mouse model. *Angiology,* 2011, 62(2), 144-154. doi: 10.1177/0003319710387919.

Parikh, A; Childress, C; Deitrick, K; Lin, Q; Rukstalis, D; Yang, W. Statin-induced autophagy by inhibition of geranylgeranyl biosynthesis in prostate cancer PC3 cells. *Prostate,* 2010, 70(9), 971-981. doi: 10.1002/pros.21131.

Pislar, A; Kos, J. Cysteine cathepsins in neurological disorders. *Mol. Neurobiol.*, 2014, 49(2): 1017-1030.

Qian, C; Wei, B; Ding, J; Wu, H; Cai, X; Li, B; Wang, Y. Meta-analysis comparing the effects of rosuvastatin versus atorvastatin on regression of coronary atherosclerotic plaques. *Am. J. Cardiol.*, 2015, 116(10): 1521-1526. doi: 10.1016/j.amjcard.2015.08.010.

Qin, Y; Shi, GP. Cysteinyl cathepsins and mast cell proteases in the pathogenesis and therapeutics of cardiovascular diseases. *Pharmacol. Ther.*, 2011, 131, 338–350.

Repnik, U; Česen, MH; Turk, B. The endolysosomal system in cell death and survival. *Cold Spring Harb Perspect. Biol.*, 2013, 5(1): a008755. doi: 10.1101/cshperspect.a008755.

Shon, SM; Choi, Y; Kim, JY; Lee, DK; Park, JY; Schellingerhout, D; Kim, DE. Photodynamic therapy using a protease-mediated theranostic agent reduces cathepsin-B activity in mouse atheromata *in vivo*. *Arterioscler. Thromb. Vasc. Biol.*, 2013, 33(6), 1360-1365.

Solberg, R; Smith, R; Almlöf, M; Tewolde, E; Nilsen, H; Johansen, HT. Legumain expression, activity and secretion are increased during monocyte-to-macrophage differentiation and inhibited by atorvastatin. *Biol. Chem.*, 2015, 396(1), 71-80. doi: 10.1515/hsz-2014-0172.

Stoekenbroek, RM; Boekholdt, SM; Fayyad, R; Laskey, R; Tikkanen, MJ;, Pedersen, TR; Hovingh, GK. Incremental Decrease in End Points Through Aggressive Lipid Lowering Study Group. High-dose atorvastatin is superior to moderate-dose simvastatin in preventing peripheral arterial disease. *Heart,* 2015, 101(5), 356-362. doi: 10.1136/heartjnl-2014-306906.

Stoka, V; Turk, B; Turk, V. Lysosomal cysteine proteases: structural features and their role in apoptosis. *IUBMB Life*, 2005, 57(4–5), 347–353.

Svechnikova, IG; Korolenko, TA; Stashko, JuF; Kaledin, VI; Nikolin, VP; Nowicky, JW. The influence of Ukrain on the growth of HA-1 tumor in mice: the role of cysteine proteinases as markers of tumor malignancy. *Drugs Exp. Clin. Res.,* 1998, 24(5-6), 261-269.

Tarantino, N; Santoro, F; De Gennaro, L; Correale, M; Guastafierro, F; Gaglione, A; Di Biase, M; Brunetti, ND. Fenofibrate/simvastatin fixed-dose combination in the treatment of mixed dyslipidemia: safety, efficacy, and place in therapy. *Vasc. Health Risk Manag.*, 2017,13, 29-41. doi: 10.2147/VHRM.S95044. eCollection 2017.

Toepfer, N; Childress, C; Parikh, A; Rukstalis, D; Yang, W. Atorvastatin induces autophagy in prostate cancer PC3 cells through activation of LC3 transcription. *Cancer Biol. Ther.,* 2011, 12(8), 691-699. doi: 10.4161/cbt.12.8.15978.

Turk, V; Turk, B; Turk, D. Lysosomal cysteine proteases: facts and opportunities. *Embo J.,* 2001, 20(17), 4629–4633.

Violi, F; Carnevale, R; Pastori, D; Pignatelli, P. Antioxidant and antiplatelet effects of atorvastatin by Nox2 inhibition. *Trends Cardiovasc. Med.,* 2014, 24(4), 142-148. doi: 10.1016/j.tcm.2013.09.006.

Wallin, H; Abrahamson, M; Ekström, U. Cystatin C properties crucial for uptake and inhibition of intracellular target enzymes. *J. Biol. Chem.,* 2013, 288 (23), 17 019-17 029.

Wang, W; Wang, H; Geng, QX; Wang, HT; Miao, W; Cheng, B; Zhao, D; Song, GM; Leanne, G; Zhao, Z. Augmentation of autophagy by atorvastatin via Akt/mTOR pathway in spontaneously hypertensive rats. *Hypertens Res*., 2015, 38(12), 813-820. doi: 10.1038/hr.2015.85

Wu, TC; Leu, HB; Lin, WT; Lin, CP; Lin, SJ; Chen, JW. Plasma matrix metalloproteinase-3 level is an independent prognostic factor in stable coronary artery disease. *Eur. J. Clin. Invest.,* 2005, 35(9), 537-545.

Ye, YC; Zhao, XL; Zhang, SY. Use of atorvastatin in lipid disorders and cardiovascular disease in Chinese patients. *Chin. Med. J.* (Engl), 2015, 128(2), 259-266. doi: 10.4103/0366-6999.149226.

Zarzecki, MS; Araujo, SM; Bortolotto, VC; de Paula, MT; Jesse, CR., Prigol, M. Hypolipidemic action of chrysin on Triton WR-1339-induced hyperlipidemia in female C57BL/6 mice. *Toxicology Reports,* 2014, 1, 200–208. doi: 10.1016/j.toxrep.2014.02.003. eCollection 2014.

Zhang, Q; Yang, YJ; Wang, H; Dong, QT; Wang, TJ; Qian, HY; Xu, H. Autophagy activation: a novel mechanism of atorvastatin to protect mesenchymal stem cells from hypoxia and serum deprivation via AMP-activated protein kinase/mammalian target of rapamycin pathway. *Stem Cells Dev*., 2012, 21(8), 1321-1332. doi: 10.1089/scd.2011.0684.

Zhao, X; Liu, Y; Zhong, Y; Liu, B; Yu, K; Shi, H; Zhu, R; Meng, K; Zhang, W; Wu, B; Zeng, Q. Atorvastatin Improves Inflammatory Response in Atherosclerosis by Upregulating the Expression of GARP. *Mediators Inflamm*., 2015, 2015, 841472. http://dx.doi.org/10.1155/2015/841472.

Zhu, Y; Zhang, HP; Wang, YC; Ren, TT; Li, J; Xu, ML; Wang, XQ; Liu, FC; Lau, A; Wen, YF. Serum cystatin C level is associated with carotid intima-media thickening and plaque. *Scand. J. Clin. Lab.* Invest., 2015, 75(3), 265-272.

In: Advances in Health and Disease. Volume 4 ISBN: 978-1-53613-345-5
Editor: Lowell T. Duncan

Chapter 5

FOCUS GROUPS IN HEALTH DISPARITIES RESEARCH: LESSONS LEARNED FROM AN HIV PREVENTION PROGRAM WITH HISPANIC YOUNG ADULTS

Sofia Fernandez*[*], *PhD, Rachel Clarke, PhD, Melissa Howard, PhD, Staci Morris, PsyD, Michelle Hospital, PhD and Eric F. Wagner, PhD
FIU-BRIDGE, Florida International University, Miami, FL, US

ABSTRACT

Community-based research (CBR) methods are essential for addressing the social, structural, and environmental factors that contribute to health disparities among underrepresented yet disproportionately affected minority groups. CBR enriches project implementation and the research process by involving community members in all project phases, leading to insights and health enhancements, and program sustainability

[*] Corresponding Author Email: sofernan@fiu.edu.

not otherwise obtainable. Research aimed at alleviating persistent health disparities, particularly targeting behavioral health and preventable diseases, requires deliberate and direct involvement of the population of interest in order to be most effective and promote sustained change. In CBR, key stakeholders are actively involved and engaged in the research process from the start. These stakeholders have a direct impact on the decisions made in the design, implementation, and evaluation of projects. Conducting focus groups can be an effective way to involve the population of interest in the research process. Focus groups give community members the opportunity to recount experiences, share insights, and engage in dialogue with other community members and the researchers with whom they are partnering. Focus groups can be particularly helpful when dealing with racial, ethnic or sexual minority groups, whose experiences often do not mirror the experiences of those from the dominant culture. Furthermore, focus groups can inform researchers about how specific minority subgroups of individuals receive and exchange health information that they find credible and impactful. Such knowledge is critical for the successful dissemination of health information using social media and networking technologies, given the fast pace of change and the immense popularity of these communication tools among young adults. Focus groups can help ensure that the needs of underrepresented and rapidly changing populations are understood, that projects are culturally and linguistically appropriate and relevant, and that trust and communication between researchers and community members is established and maintained. This chapter describes focus groups conducted as part of a federally-funded University CBR partnership program for preventing HIV and substance abuse among Hispanic emerging adults in Miami-Dade County. Miami-Dade County has the highest rates of HIV infection in the U. S. Using a real-world example, this chapter will discuss how employing focus groups provided the opportunity to 1) check cultural assumptions, 2) assess and prioritize areas of greatest perceived need, 3) tailor campaigns and outreach to the key values and beliefs of population of focus, and 4) understand and capitalize on social media and other communication favored by the population of focus to reduce health disparities. This chapter also offer suggestions as to how focus groups can be used as an instrumental technique to contributing to the success of CBR partnerships aimed at promoting health equity and alleviating health disparities, specifically related to HIV, among minority communities.

Keywords: community-based research partnership, ethnic minority, young adults, HIV prevention, communication technologies

COMMUNITY-BASED RESEARCH

The importance of formative research when addressing health disparities among underrepresented, underserved, disproportionally affected communities cannot be overstated. In order to create successful lasting improvements in community health, researchers need to understand the communities they are serving and the conditions these communities need to be healthy (Minkler, Garcia, Rubin, & Wallerstein, 2012). Community partners provide an understanding of the issues faced by community members, the culture of the local community, and how community issues and culture together may impact the health and well-being of community members. Health disparities research, in particular, requires deliberate and direct involvement of the population of interest in order to be as effective as it can be and to promote sustained enhancements. Community-based research (CBR) was long ago defined as "a collaborative approach to research that equitably involves, for example, community members, organizational representatives, and researchers in all aspects of the research process" (Israel, Schulz, Parker, & Becker, 1998, p. 177). This definition has remained unchanged, though methods and approaches have become considerably more sophisticated over the past two decades. Still today, it is widely recognized that CBR methods are essential for addressing the social, structural, and environmental factors that contribute to health disparities among underrepresented racial and ethnic minority groups (Israel et al., 1998; Minkler & Wallerstein, 2017).

CBR can enrich project design and implementation by involving community members, especially key stakeholders, in all project phases (Minkler et al., 2012). Stakeholders -- individuals living in the community with directly relevant personal or professional knowledge and community regard-- can identify possible barriers to implementation, as well as enhance the research design, implementation, evaluation, and interpretation-of-outcomes of projects. By conducting a comprehensive needs assessment, researchers can gain insight into what stakeholders view as the problems within the community, how they view the problem(s), and key players in the community who will be essential in finding solutions to the health problems that they face (Israel, Eng, Schulz, & Parker, 2013). Community members also can help to develop and refine study methods so they are best suited for the community being served.

Conducting focus groups can be an effective, inclusive and efficient way to involve the population of interest in the research process (Israel et al., 2013). Focus groups provide a platform for members of the community to voice their hopes and their concerns, providing valuable information to the researchers. It is essential that focus groups are conducted in familiar settings, so that community members can be comfortable engaging in convenient and convivial conversation about issues concerning them (Gilmore, 2012). Moreover, focus groups provide a setting for answering questions community members might have about the research. It is also essential that focus groups are conducted in a culturally sensitive manner, facilitating the inclusion of community members who otherwise might have been too intimidated or too busy to participate in individual interviews. Focus groups provide a nuanced understanding of the community, directly from those living in that community, as well as an in-depth understanding of broader systemic issues that may need to be addressed before progress toward health equity can be made (Kieffer et al., 2013).

A CBR Partnership

The "Miami-Dade Partnership for Preventing Health Risks among Young Adults" was a 3-year grant funded by the Substance Abuse and Mental Health Services Administration (SAMHSA, 1H79SP020653; PI: Wagner). The primary aim of the Partnership was develop and implement a culturally sensitive strategic plan for implementing HIV, Hepatitis-C and substance abuse prevention strategies for Hispanic young adults. Prevention strategies included HIV testing and counseling, as well as social media prevention and awareness campaigns. This project represented a University-Community partnership which brought together (a) a large minority serving institution (MSI) with over 50,000 students (64% Hispanic), and (b) two separate CBOs based in Miami-Dade County, FL (2.6 million persons, 64% Hispanic). The primary aim of the project was to reduce substance abuse (SA), HIV/AIDS, and hepatitis C (HCV) among Hispanic young adults (ages 18-24) in Miami-Dade through comprehensive, integrated SA, HIV and HCV prevention.

As part of the needs assessment process, researchers conducted focus groups (N = 30) with the target population (Hispanic 18-24 year olds). Participants were recruited by placing flyers at high traffic student locations around the university campus. Participants were eligible to participate if they were a) 18-24 years old b) Hispanic c) willing to provide written consent to participate. Participants were given the option of four different focus group meeting days in order to accommodate their class schedules. Focus groups met on campus at a university conference room. Participants were given a small lunch or breakfast and $10 compensation for their participation. All study protocols were approved by the Institutional Review Board of the university where the study took place.

Each focus group lasted one hour and were led by co-investigators of the primary project. Focus group leaders used a predetermined guideline, which listed key questions to initiate the discussion. An iterative CBR process was used to develop the focus group leader guide. Initially the researchers solicited feedback from the community partners involved with the project – (a) HIV testing organization administrators, (b) media consultant and (c) evaluation team. These individuals' feedback was used to develop an initial set of questions. A second round of feedback was solicited from student research associates who happened to meet the demographic profiles of the project's target population (i.e., 18-24 y/o Hispanic). This second round of feedback used to guide the final refinement of the focus group questions. Focus group leaders used this set of open ended questions solely as a guide and allowed for other conversations to unfold naturally among focus group participants, harnessing the group dynamics to benefit the depth and breadth of data collection.

Focus group participants were also given a paper survey to complete anonymously; the survey repeated key questions from the leader guide, and provided space for additional comments. Additional comments were encouraged when participants felt they had more to say than what was said in the group, wanted to keep answers private, or had other concerns or ideas that they felt more comfortable disclosing using the anonymous survey. All focus groups were audio recorded. Focus group recordings were transcribed verbatim by three transcribers.

A total of 30 18-14 y/o Hispanic students participated in the focus group sessions. Participants came from different majors ranging from social work to biology. Groups were mixed- gender. Sixty-three percent of the participants were females and 33% were male, accurately reflecting the makeup of the university student body. Half (50%) of the participants were college seniors, and 80% identified as heterosexual (10% identified as bisexual). One third (33%) of the participants were foreign born, and 67% were U. S. born. In the sections that follow, we review how findings from these focus groups informed the development, implementation and dissemination of prevention strategies for Hispanic young adults, specifically focused on reducing HIV related disparities.

Cultural and Developmental Tailoring

Health communication and educational materials that are learner-centered and culturally and linguistically appropriate for their target audience tend to have greater impacts (Resnicow et al., 2000). Strategies can be applied to program materials and messages whereby making them more appealing to a culturally distinct priority population (Kreuter et al., 2003). This may include the application of "peripheral" design elements such as images, colors, fonts or sounds—which can create interest for a given group--or linguistic elements such as providing materials in the dominant or native language of the target population. Other known strategies for enhancing cultural appropriateness include paying close attention to culture-specific conceptualizations of the health issue and through cultural targeting and tailoring (Kreuter et al., 2003). Therefore, the development of culturally sensitive prevention programs should include an analysis of epidemiological data in order to define priority groups, as well as research into the motivations and preferences related to health among members of the priority group.

Focus groups can serve exploratory functions as well as dress rehearsal functions, for example, the pre-testing program techniques and materials based on principles of health communication and social marketing (Kotler & Lee, 2016; National Cancer Institute, 2004). In the current case, we first used focus groups to explore ideas about how to adapt HIV/STI testing services, and how to design and deliver culturally sensitive HIV/STI testing information, to young Hispanic adults. We also used focus groups to pretest our program approach and materials. Stated succinctly, findings from our focus groups revealed 18-24 y/o Hispanic college students want easy-to-access HIV/STI testing and prevention services, and they want these services be normalized (as a regular part of a young adult's health routine) in order to ensure adoption and adherence to testing. Focus group participants also agreed that although print media (flyers and signs) were a viable means for advertising HIV/STI testing services and disseminating information, social media would be the most effective way to reach young adults.

Among the focus group participants, there was less consensus regarding the need and means for cultural targeting of services and messages specifically to Hispanics. Participants could not readily identify predominant phrases, or imagery that they felt would adequately represent Hispanics for the purpose of informing design concepts related to HIV prevention. Though the focus group participants represented a range of acculturation and assimilation (e.g., 33% were foreign born), the majority spoke a blend of English and Spanish in the home. Some participants suggested using bilingual materials or selected key words in Spanish might take on special meaning to grab the attention of bilingual, bicultural readers. However, there was an overwhelming consensus that English should dominate and that messages and materials should be mainly, if not entirely, in English.

In South Florida, Hispanics are a majority-minority group, and thus proportionally the largest racial/ethnic group. However, South Florida

Hispanics are better described not as a single group but as multiple subgroups, representing multiple countries of origin and unique cultures from Latin America and the Caribbean. Though the largest portion of Hispanics in South Florida report Cuban heritage, Florida Hispanics have roots in Puerto Rico, Colombia, Nicaragua, Venezuela, Mexico and other South and Central American countries (U.S. Census Bureau, 2010). As noted by the focus group participants, the labels “Hispanic” or “Latino” were perceived as constricting and uninformative, disregarding the unique cultures, ethnicities, races, and countries of origin that make up a Hispanic person’s background. This observation of our focus group participants was consistent with scholar’s observations that the terms Hispanic and Latino inadequately describe the rich heterogeneity of the various populations with roots in Spanish-speaking countries (López et al., 2010).

Focus group participants largely agreed that they wanted to be acknowledged more for their generational uniqueness and developmental life stage (i.e., young adulthood) than for their Hispanic identity. As a result, program design elements that highlighted participants’ millennial statuses, were more appealing than program design elements that highlighted participants’ Hispanic backgrounds. Furthermore, participants were attracted to communication strategies relying on the use of social media and were attentive to information about non-stigmatizing behavioral prevention strategies, which could easily be fit into daily routines and performed quickly.

Focus groups were also used for pre-testing, during which members of the target audience were exposed to materials and messages for the purpose of obtaining feedback prior to program launch (National Cancer Institute, 2004). In the current study, researchers presented participants with conceptual elements of the intervention and asked them to comment on specific messages, artwork, or intervention themes, in order to home cultural and linguistic appropriateness and appeal. Such pre-testing is particularly important when a behavior or disease is associated with social stigma, as are HIV related risk behaviors (Resnicow et al., 2000). Pre-test feedback from focus groups proved to be very helpful to the program planners and provided insights into target audience perceptions of program components.

It is important to acknowledge that cultural and linguistic sensitivity is best practiced when culture-specific conceptualizations of the health issue—which may be more heavily influenced by lifestyle, preferences, opinions and personality characteristics— are additionally taken into consideration. Historically, many HIV/STI prevention programs targeting young adults have not been sensitive in this manner. Cultural sensitivity should at the very least be considered during the needs assessment and pre-testing phases of health promotion programs targeting underrepresented, underserved minority populations. In addition, inclusion of community members in all phases of program design would further ensure cultural and linguistic sensitivity, relevance, and appeal.

Although focus groups can be instrumental in meeting a wide range of research goals, the functions and capabilities of focus groups are especially advantageous when dealing with racial and ethnic minority groups, whose experiences do not mirror the experiences of those from the dominant culture. Focus groups can help ensure that the needs of the targeted population are understood, that projects are culturally and linguistically appropriate and relevant, and that trust and communication between researchers and community members is established and maintained. Focus groups are a valuable tool to elicit feedback from underrepresented populations, as well as to keep up with rapidly changing societal and personal trends influencing health promotion and disease prevention efforts.

Social Media Based Strategies in HIV Prevention

The efforts of the present CBR partnership included traditional HIV prevention risk reduction strategies and the promotion of evidenced-based behaviors. We provided free HIV/ STI rapid testing services on campus (offered through the grass-roots, community based service providers) and distributed and promoted female and male condoms. However, structural barriers, including limited access to relevant information about available prevention services for minority young adults, were also identified and addressed in program strategies. Partnership efforts included increasing access to tailored and relevant health information in a convenient and credible manner.

Chronic underutilization of sexual health services by ethnic minority young adults speaks to the need for culturally and linguistically tailored and developmentally engaging programs for this population. Health equity cannot be achieved without such population-specific tailoring and presentation. Because of the ubiquitous use of and enthusiastic preference for social media communication technologies among our focus group participants, as well the ability of social media for widespread reach, our program incorporated a heavy emphasis on social media communication technologies.

Social media is an umbrella term that encompasses a range of web technologies where users create, share and or exchange information and ideas in virtual communities (Smith & Denali, 2014). Social networking sites are a type of social media that are distinguished by the unique ability for users to construct a public profile and to form a list of users with whom they share a connection (Boyd & Ellison, 2010). Social networking sites are the most popular forms of social media among young adults and, today, the most commonly used social networking platform is Facebook. In fact, Facebook is the most popular website nationwide after Google and YouTube (Alexa Internet, Inc., 2017).

Power differences and communication gaps present as barriers in the development and adoption of effective programs for underserved and underrepresented minorities. A key characteristic and standard in CBR is the commitment to shared power and resources (Horowitz, Robinson, & Seifer, 2009). Implementing prevention messaging through a social media campaign— a space where focus group participants reported active and preferred communication—allowed us to minimize barriers to relevant information and maximize feedback and involvement from the population of focus. Researchers harnessed the interactive nature of social media based technologies by encouraging users to respond, ask questions, express opinions, and be a part of their community's health conversations (Ems & Gonzalez, 2016). Utilizing social media based strategies underscored principles upheld in the CBR partnership and provided an opportunity for a communication space which encompassed opportunities for enhanced access to information, as well as social and community support and connection.

Focus Groups as Enhancement of Social Media Understanding

Through the use of focus groups, researchers enhanced their understanding of using social media technologies in health communication with young adults and also received critical information that guided the implementation of both online and offline efforts in necessary ways.

Although, in the literature, the most researched social networking site continues to be Facebook, our focus groups participants identified Instagram as the most popularly used social networking site among their community, with Twitter as the second most popular. This is consistent with a recent Pew Research study examining social networking trends among ethnic minority young adults; Hispanics and African Americans were more likely to report using Instagram than were non-Hispanic Whites (Krogstad, 2015).

Successfully engaging minority young adults online can be a challenging task. Rapidly changing functionalities of social networking sites continually shift the way users communicate online and which particular sites are most popular at any given time. This mercurial quality speaks to the risks inherent in solely relying on the available published literature, which inherently and inevitably lags behind current trends in social networking uses. Furthermore, different social networking sites have different languages, slang words, and tones from one another, complicating direct comparisons across sites. Ensuring that content and messaging is culturally and linguistically appropriate in tone and style is critical in engaging young minority adults online. Focus groups allowed researchers to understand appropriate and contemporary uses of social networking sites in their targeted community, as well threats and barriers to the credibility and utility of online communications. For example, focus groups findings revealed that "tagging" or linking a personal account with prevention campaign material (something we were considering doing) would violate trust and harm the relationship between the CBR team and the young adult community. Needless to say, our focus group findings led us to drop the idea of tagging as part of our social media campaign.

Lessons Learned in Utilizing Social Media Based Strategies

This CBR partnership utilized Instagram, Twitter, and Facebook, as social media avenues to enhance dissemination of health promotion content. By providing relevant information about locally available services and by providing health tips in the form of brief, online social networking posts, this CBR partnership used social media to increase access to HIV prevention information and services expressly designed for Hispanic young adults.

Our work has demonstrated that, in order to promote sustained community engagement online, social media messaging must be timely, developmentally appropriate (in tone and style), and culturally and linguistically appropriate. The CBR partnership used a social media campaign to deliver information about testing services that were actively and locally available by posting updates in real time (3 times per week on average). The CBR partnership also utilized formative feedback from focus group participants to develop and disseminate non-threatening and normalizing health education about HIV risk and sexual health promotion. Our work further suggests volunteers who have active roles in prevention programming offline (e.g., as recruiters at health fairs) should leverage their experiences and clout to serve as a connection between online and offline efforts.

HIV prevention researchers have a responsibility to provide information and services that are specific to vulnerable and high risk populations. Choosing communication strategies that complement the daily routines and realities of individuals in high risk groups is a deliberate step that can be taken by researchers in order to increase message acceptance and adoption. The incorporation of authentic and appropriate messaging online with underserved and underrepresented minority young adults will enhance trust and, thus, improve the recruitment and retention of disproportionately affected minority populations in HIV prevention services.

The efforts of the CBR partnership confirmed that sexual health topics have a place online to which young adults give attention. Social media technologies allow for new opportunities in communication among public health researchers, community based service providers, other professionals, and populations in need of services, as well as for new metrics by which to estimate the impact of social media campaigns. Based on focus group findings and the implementation and preliminary evaluation of the social media campaign, we found that integrating social media based efforts into a larger prevention campaign (e.g., posters, billboards, and classroom presentations) was particularly effective. Social media campaigns should not be launched in isolation, but rather should be a synergistic part of a larger, more comprehensive prevention program. In our focus groups, when the topic of social media was introduced, participants supported its use across various platforms, but also stated a desire for "old-fashioned" flyers in high traffic areas, pointing out that these formats were more tangible and less easily forgotten. Focus group participants also desired an in-person presence prior to and during events and settings often associated with high risk behaviors (e.g., tailgating, homecoming, spring break).

We found focus groups to be a valuable tool to gain information about optimal ways to use social media to promote health among young adult Hispanic college students. Focus groups provided a direct opportunity for researchers to gather contemporary information on rapidly changing communication technologies, and thus leapfrog the considerable lag found in published research. Furthermore, using social media for ongoing formative feedback about our prevention campaign was possible by posting questions, soliciting ideas, and encouraging participants' messaging. This helped researchers gather continual and real-time feedback about reported barriers to service adoption beyond the formative research phase.

Implementation and Dissemination

In this study, focus group findings were immediately utilized to customize and tailor the implementation and dissemination of planned HIV/STI testing services. The findings also shaped our accompanying social media campaign in order to maximize reach to our targeted population of Hispanic young adults aged 18-24. In their review of organizational health service delivery, Greenhalgh et al., (2004) favored a process orientation that focuses more on the features that contribute to a program's success than the overall evaluation of program success, especially within a particular setting. From this perspective, focusing on the unique characteristics of a particular setting has the potential to provide rich information about how or why a program succeeds or fails. To this end, our recruitment strategies, outreach events, and the social media plan were tweaked according to the findings of the focus groups, whose members represented the target audience.

Although the actual testing services were implemented according to unaltered and current CDC guidelines, our focus groups provided population- and setting-specific insights into how best to disseminate information about the widespread need for testing, availability of testing services, details of the testing procedure, and the specific days, times, and locations for testing days. Incorporating focus group feedback helped us stylize our communication and outreach strategies to best reach the targeted population, overcome barriers such as the stigma surrounding HIV/STI testing (especially among Hispanic young adults), and provide relevant and practical information on harm reduction and health promotion. A majority of focus group participants stated the need to normalize testing, remove the stigma associated with getting tested, and encourage personal responsibility for knowing one's status. Thus, an integral component of our campaign became encouraging everyone to get tested, not just "high risk" groups such as IV drug users or those who are more sexually active. As one focus group participant stated in regard to normalization of HIV testing, "It's like having a driver's license, but for sex." This resulted in environmental prevention strategies (e.g., social media posts, palm cards) encouraging everyone to

"Know your status," know the status of partner(s), and participate in easy, convenient, and free on-campus testing.

Moreover, our Hispanic young adult participants clearly stated they did not merely want to see statistics, but desired posts and messages that were supportive, not fear-based (e.g., "no scare tactics;" "HIV is not a death sentence"), and used real stories with relatable people. Some participants added that, if statistics were presented, they should be clear and not open to interpretation. As one participant stated, "We're in college. We like black and white. If we have more subjective things, we don't think it applies to us."

Focus group participants overwhelmingly indicated that privacy was key in decision-making regarding HIV testing, explaining that simply knowing why testing is important is useless without information about how and where to get tested. While a mobile testing van was available and offered, most participants stated that they would prefer a less conspicuous and more permanent place for testing; as a result, we now provide testing in inconspicuous and easily accessible ground floor offices. Focus group participants also encouraged us to emphasize in our communications that HIV testing is free, confidential/private, and brief (20 minutes). To assist interested HIV test takers to easily find the location, participants suggested easily identifiable directional signs be placed in central high traffic areas on campus.

Health researchers agree that "cultural factors…are pervasive and fundamental considerations," (Durlak & DuPre, 2008) and "the process of dissemination (in this case, spreading the word about HIV testing services) needs to be tailored to various audiences" (Brownson, 2016). However, these cultural factors are not always obvious, as focus group findings revealed. When asked about tailoring HIV prevention messages to Hispanic/Latinos, our focus group participants warned against stereotyping (don't use "people playing soccer") and recommended flyers be printed in English and Spanish on reverse sides (."..because I can read English too...and then you give me the Spanish one, it's like what? If it's flippable, then it's perfect because then...there's no [language] assumption needed").

Participants responded positively towards risk reduction messages, acknowledging that people will have sex, and some will choose to drink alcohol and/or use drugs while having sex, so messages about how to do so safely would be useful. When asked about substance use messages, participants warned against using exaggerated messaging (i.e., "one shot will not make you pass out"). They were positively inclined towards harm reduction messages, such as understanding one's drinking limits and practical suggestions such as alternating alcoholic drinks with water.

Regarding implementation at outreach events, participants stated the need for giveaways and promotional items with testing information, such as condoms. This would not only help draw an audience to tabling events, but would encourage them to actually take something away that they could use and that also provided useful information. Free condoms included the community based organizations' service information. As far as staffing, focus group participants indicated they would prefer to interact with other students and/or respected and likeable faculty and staff more so than celebrities.

A notable outcome of the focus groups was a clear consensus on the best day to conduct testing. Participants overwhelmingly endorsed Wednesday, also known as "hump day" as the ideal day for HIV testing. The idea stimulated a very productive brainstorming session among the group members and the idea for a camel (with a hump) mascot emerged. This important focus group finding was integral in the creation of the environmental outreach and social media campaign using "Cody the Camel," a genderless, identifiable character with a name that was pronounced well in both English and Spanish, and had a clever association to the campaign. Cody the Camel promotes free, confidential HIV/STI testing on Wednesday "hump" days, and gives useful tips for safer "turn ups" (i.e., harm-reduction tips on how to party more safely), through a print and social media environmental prevention plan.

Focus group findings were shared with members of the project's Community Advisory Board, collegiate and local stakeholders who assisted in the refinement of materials and made suggestions for improvement. These suggestions often included partnering with other key stakeholders, both individuals and groups, on campus with common and related goals to support each other's health promotion and risk reduction efforts. The implementation of this project was not only a research project, but also served to bridge the gap between scientific findings and dissemination of those findings to a larger population.

The dissemination of information regarding the importance and need for HIV testing for "everyone," and the implementation of the suggestions provided by focus group participants who assisted in the development of the social media and environmental outreach campaign proved to be successful, as evidenced by the number of tests conducted, and even more so by the number of first-time tests (over 1,600 total tests to 18-24 year old Hispanics between September 2015 and April 2017, of which, approximately half were tested for the first time). Dissemination and implementation (D&I) models or frameworks are becoming increasingly popular, and useful, in the field of health research, programming, and evaluation (Tabak, et al., 2012) and have promise to increase capacity for health promotion service provision in the community (Glasgow et. al, 2012). D&I is a process to facilitate "bridging the gap" between research and real-world settings (Durlak & DuPre, 2008). Dissemination, broadly speaking, refers to the process of providing information and materials to a targeted population, "public health, or clinical audience" (Glasgow et. al, 2012; Brownson, 2016). This information is usually clinical or health-based in nature and is often evidence-based. Implementation is the use of strategies to facilitate program adoption and bring health-based intervention, and often evidence-based intervention, to communities to improve client health and outcomes (Glasgow et. al, 2012; Brownson, 2016).

Through this CBR partnership and the use of focus groups, we gained valuable feedback about the ways in which using social media strategies mat be most effective for 18-24 year old Hispanic young adults in South Florida. In order to increase acceptance and adoption, researchers implemented focus groups to gain feedback on the types of messaging for prevention content, the types of social media platforms that would be most appropriate to deliver this content, and the ways in which to link or not link individuals with this HIV prevention information online.

The focus group findings directly affected the project implementation and served to bridge the gaps between the grant investigators, the service providers, and the population of focus towards achieving the goal of alleviating health disparities. While the actual testing procedures were scientifically sound, accurate, and quick, there was a clear need to develop more effective methods of "getting the word out" and reaching the hardest to reach, most vulnerable people. Focus groups also served as a valuable tool to stay abreast to the rapidly involving and growing potential of social media as a tool in HIV prevention communication with Hispanic young adults. Utilizing focus groups with representatives of the target population and consulting with key stakeholders served to build administrative support within the university and build capacity for the implementation of this type of program. This formative phase not only allowed for, but encouraged flexibility and refinements along the way, in order to overcome barriers and facilitate service provision and the promotion of healthier behaviors. Future studies could focus on maintenance of the services provided, periodically utilize additional focus groups to gather fresh ideas and stay current, gather data on the long-term implications to the university to gain and maintain support, and utilize a dissemination and implementation model for evaluation.

REFERENCES

Alexa Internet, Inc. (2017). The top 500 sites on the web. *An Amazon Company.* Retrieved from https://www.alexa.com/topsites.

Boyd, D., & Ellison, N. (2010). Social network sites: definition, history, and scholarship. *IEEE Engineering Management Review*, *3*(38), 16-31.

Brownson, R. C. (2016). *Dissemination Science & Designing for Dissemination* [PowerPoint slides]. Presented for Training Institute for Dissemination And Implementation Research in Health Introduction Webinar.

Casado, B. L., Negi, N. J., & Hong, M. (2012). Culturally competent social work research: Methodological considerations for research with language minorities. *Social Work*, *57*(1), 1-10.

Durlak, J. A. and DuPre, E. P. (2008). Implementation matters: A review of research on the influence of implementation on program outcomes and the factors affecting implementation. *American Journal of Community Psychology*, 41, 327–350. Doi: 10.1007/s10464-008-9165-0.

Ems, L., & Gonzales, A. L. (2016). Subculture-centered public health communication: A social media strategy. *New Media & Society*, *18*(8), 1750-1767.

Gilmore, G. D. (2012). *Needs and Capacity Assessment Strategies for Health Education and Health Promotion*. Burlington, MA: Jones & Bartlett Learning.

Glasgow, R. E., Vinson, C., Chambers, D., Khoury, M. J., Kaplan, R. M., & Hunter, C. (2012). National Institutes of Health approaches to dissemination and implementation science: Current and future directions. *American Journal of Public Health*, 102 (7), 1274-1281. doi: 10.2105/AJPH.2012.300755.

Greenhalgh, T., Robert, G., Macfarlane, F., Bate, P., & Kyriakidou, O. (2004). Diffusion of innovations in service organizations: Systematic review and recommendations. *Milbank Quarterly*, 82, 581–629. doi:10.1111/j.0887.

Horowitz, C. R., Robinson, M., & Seifer, S. (2009). Community-based participatory research from the margin to the mainstream. *Circulation*, *119*(19), 2633-2642.

Israel, B. A., Schulz, A. J., Parker, E. A., & Becker, A. B. (1998). Review of community-based research: assessing partnership approaches to improve public health. *Annual Review of Public Health*, *19*(1), 173-202.

Israel, B. A., Eng, E., Schulz, A. J., & Parker, E. A. (2013) *Methods for community-based participatory research for health*. San Fancisco, CA: Jossey-Bass.

Kieffer, E. C., Salabarria-Pena, Y., Odoms-Young, A. M., Willis, S. K., Palmisano, G., & Guzman, J. R. (2013). The application of focus group methodologies to CBPR. In B. A. Israel, E. Eng, A. J. Schulz, & E. A.

Parker (Eds.), *Methods for Community-based Participatory Research for Health* (pp. 249-276). San Fancisco, CA: Jossey-Bass.

Kotler, N. & Lee, P. (2016). *Social Marketing: Changing Behaviors for Good* (5th ed). Sage: Thousand Oaks, CA.

Kreuter, M., Lukwago, S., Bucholtz, D., Clark, E. & Sanders-Thompson, V. (2003). Achieving Cultural Appropriateness in Health Promotion Programs: Targeted and Tailored Approaches. *Health Education & Behavior*, 30 (2), 133-146.

Krogstad, J. (2015). *Social media preferences vary by race and ethnicity. Pew Research Center*. Retrieved from http://www.pewresearch.org /fact-tank/2015/02/03/social-media-preferences-vary-by-race-and-ethnicity/.

López, E., Morales, G., Saucedo, C., Aguirre-Girón L., Mack, S. & Goodkin, K. (2010). A proposition against using the terms "Hispanic" and "Latino" in research on HIV-associated neurocognitive disorders. *Ethnicity & Disease*, *20*, 479–484.

Minkler, M., Garcia, A. P., Rubin, V., & Wallerstein, N. (2012). *Community-based participatory research: A strategy for building healthy communities and promoting health through policy change.* Oakland: PolicyLink.

Minkler, M., & Wallerstein, N. (2017). *Community-based participatory research for health: From process to outcomes* (3rd ed.). San Francisco, CA: Jossey-Bass.

National Cancer Institute. (2004). *Making Health Communication Programs Work: A Planner's Guide*. U. S. Dept. of Health and Human Services, National Institutes of Health, [Office of Cancer Communications, National Cancer Institute].

Resnicow, K., Soler, R., Braithwaite, R., Ahluwalia, J., Butler, J. (2000). Cultural Sensitivity in Substance Abuse Prevention. *Journal of Community Psychology,* 28(3), 271–290.

Smith, M., & Denali, D. (2014). Social media in health education, promotion, and communication: Reaching rural Hispanic populations along the USA/Mexico border region. *Journal of Racial and Ethnic Health Disparities, 1*(3), 194.

Tabak, R. G., Khoong, E. C., Chambers, D. A., & Brownson, R. C. (2012). Bridging research and practice: Models for dissemination and implementation research. *American Journal of Preventive Medicine*, 43 (3), 337-350. doi.org/10.1016/j.amepre.2012.05.024.

U.S. Census Bureau (2010*). 2010 Census, Community Facts*. Retrieved from: https://factfinder.census.gov/faces/nav/jsf/pages/index.xhtml

In: Advances in Health and Disease. Volume 4 ISBN: 978-1-53613-345-5
Editor: Lowell T. Duncan

Chapter 6

Congenital Hypothyroidism (CH): The Re-Evaluation of Diagnosis in CH Patients with *in Situ* Glands Identified by Newborn Screening

***R. Ortolano*[1], *M. Bitelli*[2], *F. Baronio*[1] *and A. Cassio*[2,*]**

[1]Department of Women, Child Health and Urologic Diseases, Pediatric Unit, S.Orsola-Malpighi University Hospital, Bologna, Italy
[2]Department of Medical and Surgical Sciences, Pediatric Unit, University of Bologna, Bologna, Italy

Abstract

Background: Congenital Hypothyroidism (CH) is the most common endocrine disorder in childhood. Levothyroxine treatment within the first 2-3 weeks of life prevent neurological damage. Newborn screening (NS) by TSH dosage on dried blood spot allowed to early identification of risk for CH. In the last years the reduction of TSH recall threshold has led to an

* Corresponding Author Email: alessandra.cassio@unibo.it.

increased detection of mild forms with in situ gland at the first diagnosis. Therefore, the re-evaluation of diagnosis has become an important procedure to distingue transient forms from permanent ones.

Aetiology: Transient CH may be caused by maternal factors (deficiency/excess of iodine, TSH receptor blockers, drugs) or neonatal factors (preterm and NICU infants; heterozygous mutations of the DUOX2 and DUOXA2 genes).

Epidemiology: Before NS, the incidence of CH was 1:7000-10000 live births. After the introduction of NS it increased to 1:3000-4000. Currently, it is 1:1600-2800. This increase is correlated with the lowering TSH recall threshold, the increase in multiple pregnancies and preterm infants, and demographic changes.

Re-evaluation of CH: it is performed after third year of life. According to the European guidelines, two different strategies can be adopted: the discontinuation of therapy over a period of 4-6 weeks or by decreasing the dose of Levothyroxine by 30% for 2–3 weeks followed by the dosing of serum levels of TSH and fT4. CH is permanent if an increase in TSH $\geq$ 10 mU/L is demonstrated.

The etiology of CH can be identified using thyroid ultrasound (US), Iodine-123 scintigraphy, and in selected cases the perchlorate test.

If the US shows a normal thyroid volume and scintigraphy shows low/absent tracer uptake, TSH resistance is presumable.

If the US shows a normal or increased volume of thyroid, with a greedy absorption of the tracer to scintigraphy, dyshormonogenesis by the perchlorate test could be investigated. A radiolabel wash out of 10% of baseline uptake 2 hours after administration of perclorate is indicative of a defect in organification (partial with a wash out between 10-90%; total with a wash out >90%).

The US findings of a normal or increased thyroid volume associated with high TSH and very low/unmeasurable thyroglobulin levels point to a deficiency of thyroglobulin synthesis.

In our regional program of NS in the last ten years 491/454024 children were recalled for TSH and the diagnosis of CH was confirmed in 82.5%. The incidence of CH was 1:1121 births. 280 patients showed CH with *in situ* gland. After re-evaluation of diagnosis a permanent form of CH was detected in 55% of the cases (29% with hyperthyrotropinemia).

A partial form of organification defect was detected in 34.5% of subjects submitted to perchlorate test and a TSH resistance due to a heterozygous mutation of the TSH-receptor gene was detected in 28.6%.

Birth at term, the thyroid hypoplasia and a higher therapeutic dose of Levothyroxine (>2 mcg/Kg) at the re-evaluation were predictive factors of a permanent form.

The frequent persistence of thyroid dysfunction in patients with borderline TSH values at the NS underlines the importance of reducing the recall threshold.

1. Introduction

Congenital hypothyroidism (CH) is the most common endocrine disorder in the pediatric age-group and the most frequent preventable cause of severe mental retardation [1]. It is defined as a deficiency in the thyroid hormones at birth. The beginning of levothyroxine (L-T4) replacement therapy within the first 2-3 weeks of life prevents neurological damage [2]. Newborn screening (NS) by TSH dosage on dried blood spots (DBS) leads to the early identification and therapy of subjects at risk for primary CH, thus it is possible to diagnose CH in the early days of life and to start treatment very early [3, 4].

In the last years, a reduction in the TSH recall threshold [5-7] has led to an increase in the incidence of CH, attributable largely to mild forms with in situ gland [5, 7]. Given the increased number of these cases, it is important to evaluate whether these are transient or permanent forms. Permanent CH refers to a persistent thyroid hormone deficiency requiring replacement therapy for life in patients with dysgenetic or *in situ* thyroid. Transient CH is a temporary deficit of thyroid hormones, identified at birth but then followed by the return to a condition of euthyroidism in the first months or years of life in patients with *in situ* gland. Lastly, a new nosographic entity is represented by persistent hyperthyrotropinemia, a condition characterized by a serum concentration of TSH between 5 and 10 mU/L and normal fT4 levels for age. Even if we know several causes of persistent hyperthyrotropinemia, the etiology is not always identified. This condition always requires follow-up and discussion with the family for the need or not of substitutive therapy.

The distinction between transient and permanent forms is possible through a re-evaluation of the diagnosis, generally performed after 2-3 years of age with a reduction or suspension of substitutive treatment [8-10].

2. Aetiology of Primary CH

Regarding permanent CH, in about 60% of cases the defect involves the development or migration of the thyroid gland and is thus defined as thyroid dysgenesis, while the other 40% of cases show a eutopic thyroid gland with a normal or increased volume [11]. There are three major forms of dysgenesis: thyroid ectopy, athyreosis and hypoplasia. Thyroid ectopy refers to an ectopic location of the gland, above or below the hyoid bone or above the thyroid cartilage. It is common in these cases to find a thyroid remnant along the pathway of the thyroglossal duct [12, 13]. The term athyreosis denotes the complete absence of thyroid tissue. Thyroid hypoplasia refers to a thyroid gland of reduced volume for age [14].

Thyroid dysgenesis is usually sporadic, however a genetic component is found in about 2% of cases [15]. The genes involved as a cause of thyroid dysgenesis encode for transcription factors expressed both during thyroid embryogenesis and later in the normal functioning gland. The permanent forms with *in situ* gland are due to defects in one of the steps of thyroid hormone synthesis (dyshormonogenesis), usually inherited as an autosomal recessive defect. The mutations regard different genes, encoding for the sodium-iodide symporter (NIS), thyroperoxidase (TPO), the thyroid oxidase and dual oxidase maturation factors (*DUOX2* and *DUOXA2* genes), thyroglobulin (Tg), iodothyronine deiodinases, and the transmembrane protein pendrin. Pendrin is a chloride-iodide transporter both in the thyroid and in the inner ear, and when genetically altered, it causes Pendred's syndrome, which is characterized by hypothyroidism with goiter and deafness [16]. In a minor number of cases, permanent primary CH may also be caused by mutations in the TSH receptor gene (TSH-R) or in the alpha subunit of the stimulatory guanine nucleotide binding protein (Gs alpha), both altering the TSH signal [17, 18].

Transient forms of CH can be caused by maternal or neonatal factors. All these transient cases show a thyroid gland of a normal or increased volume in its usual cervical location.

Maternal factors:

- exposure to iodine deficiency or excess (drugs or iodine antiseptic compounds);
- transplacental passage of TSH receptor blocking antibodies;
- use of antithyroid medications.

Neonatal factors:

- neonatal iodine deficiency [19] or excess;
- congenital liver hemangiomas (with increased deiodinase type 3 activity) [20];
- mutations of the heterozygous *DUOX2* and *DUOXA2* genes (partial defects in the organification of iodine) [21, 22];
- preterm infants and infants admitted to neonatal intensive care units (NICU) (twins, VLBW, critical illnesses).

Transient neonatal hypothyroidism is more frequently observed in iodine-deficient than in iodine-sufficient areas [23]. A study from an iodine-deficient area in Poland has shown that the incidence of transient congenital hypothyroidism decreased significantly after the initiation of an iodine supplementation program [24]. Primary prevention of permanent CH may be possible by ensuring an adequate nutritional iodine intake in the population. In Italy a voluntary nationwide salt iodization program was implemented in 2005 [25].

Prematurity is a risk factor for CH, both for the transient and the permanent form. Transient CH in a premature infant may result from a temporary thyroid imbalance, which may relate to hormone biosynthesis [26] or the ability to adapt to external iodine supply variations. Because the ability of the thyroid to escape the Wolff-Chaikoff effect does not mature before 36 weeks of gestation, preterm infants are at risk of exposure to excess iodine due to the topical application of iodinated antiseptics [7]. In addition, neonates admitted to NICU and subjected to parenteral nutrition (PN) present lower thyroid iodine deposits, because PN does not seem to guarantee the adequate daily intake of iodine (30 mg/kg/day) [27].

3. Epidemiology

Before NS, the diagnosis of CH only took place after the appearance of clinical manifestations. At that time, the estimated incidence was about 1: 7000-10000 live births [28, 29]. The introduction of screening programs has led to early diagnosis of the disease and therefore prevention of complications, but has also provided the opportunity to diagnose more cases of CH. In 1979 Fisher et al. reported an incidence of CH of about 1: 3000 and 1: 4000 births (data obtained from the analysis of a million newborn babies screened in the USA) [3]. This rate of incidence remained relatively constant until the 1990s when it increased in Europe, USA and other parts of the world. The incidence of CH varies between 1: 1600 and 1: 2800 according to epidemiological studies conducted in different countries (USA [30, 31], Canada [32], Greece [6], Italy [5, 20], New Zealand [33], Australia [34]). The estimated incidence in Italy is about 1: 1940 [11]. Data on the incidence in Italy are recorded in the Italian National Registry of Infants with CH (INRICH), a population-based registry that performs nationwide surveillance of CH [35].

Several factors have been proposed to explain this increase in the incidence of CH.

3.1. Changes in NS Strategy

By setting the micromethod for TSH dosing on capillary blood, most of the screening programs that used a thyroxine dosage test have shifted to a strategy based on blood-spot TSH measurements [4, 36], with increased sensitivity to the detection of mild forms. In Italy currently all screening centers use TSH on DBS as a primary test [11].

The reduction in the recall threshold for TSH, has also led to the diagnosis of many more cases of mild CH, often with thyroid *in situ*. In fact, it became evident in some screening programs that some cases of CH were escaping early diagnosis. The subjects in question only received a diagnosis later on the appearance of signs and clinical symptoms or after performing thyroid tests for familiarity [6].

3.2. Preterm and NICU Infants

Prematurity is a risk factor for CH, both for the transient and the permanent forms. Between 1987-2008 in Italy, preterm infants represented 12.4% of newborn infants with permanent CH and 30.7% of those with transient CH. These percentages were particularly high in view of the fact that only 6.5% of the Italian neonatal population born between 1987 and 2008 were preterm infants [11]. Improvements in perinatal and neonatal care have since significantly increased the survival rate of preterm infants [37]. The increased survival of premature neonates, a higher category of risk for CH, has certainly contributed to increasing the incidence of this disease.

3.3. Multiple Pregnancies

In the last few decades, due to the greater use of assisted reproduction techniques and induced ovulation drugs, there has been an increase in multiple births [38, 39]. In twins, the risk of CH is three times higher than in infants born from single pregnancies.

3.4. Demographic Changes

The incidence of CH may also be affected by changes in the ethnic composition of the population as a result of migration flows. The risk of congenital hypothyroidism seems to be different in different ethnicities. Between 1991 and 2000 in the United States Hinton et al. reported a greater frequency of CH in white babies, but an even greater frequency in Hispanic and Asian infants [41]. The increase in migration of some ethnic groups characterized by a higher risk of CH and also a high fertility rate in Western countries, could therefore contribute to the incidence of CH in these countries. Moreover, the prevalence of births from consanguineous parents should be considered in the different ethnic groups. According to Olivieri et al., between 1987 and 2008 the rate of consanguinity was found to be considerably higher in Italy among African babies (24%), Asians (13%) and Hispanics (9%) compared to Caucasian infants (2%) [11]. Of the babies with CH born to consanguineous parents, the frequency of *in situ* thyroid is significantly higher compared to thyroid dysgenesis (65 vs 35%). This suggests a high recurrence of genetic dyshormonogenesis in this category of patients [11].

4. Diagnosis Confirmation

According to guidelines [8], positive screening results are confirmed by definitive tests of serum thyroid function. These include TSH and free T4, whose concentrations are considered normal when included in the age-related reference intervals available in the literature [26]. Thyroid ultrasound and/or scintigraphy are generally performed to complete the diagnosis with information on aetiology and severity of CH. Infants with positive screening results are therefore referred to a follow-up center to confirm the diagnosis and to start replacement therapy. At the time of diagnosis, besides the biochemical analysis of TSH and fT4 serum concentrations, a complete anamnesis is collected in all patients and a careful clinical examination performed, looking for early signs of CH, such as prolonged neonatal jaundice (lasting more than 72hrs), dry skin, cold extremities, macroglossia, umbilical hernia, sleepiness, poor and slow feeding, hypotonia, large anterior, and posterior fontanelles [8, 9].

5. Re-Evaluation of Diagnosis in CH Patients with *in situ* Thyroid Gland

CH patients with *in situ* thyroid gland, who did not receive an etiologic diagnosis as neonates or in whom known causes of permanent CH were not found, should undergo a re-evaluation of the diagnosis, in order to distinguish between transient and permanent forms [8, 9].

The re-evaluation is usually performed after the age of three, because the myelination of the central nervous system, a process requiring thyroid hormones, is completed by 36 to 40 months of age (as demonstrated by magnetic resonance studies) [8]. However, if transient thyroid dysfunction is likely, the re-evaluation can be carried out earlier, after one year of age. This can happen, for example, in children with anti-thyroid antibodies detected in the blood at birth or exposed to an excess of iodine in neonatal age, or also in patients who did not need an increase in levothyroxine during the first months of life [9].

According to European guidelines [8], two different strategies for re-evaluation are possible. L-T4 should be phased out over a four to six weeks period (depending on the size of the maintenance dose) and a full re-evaluation carried out at the end of this period, with biochemical testing and thyroid imaging if hypothyroidism is confirmed. Otherwise the L-T4 dose can be decreased by 30% for two to three weeks. If during this period, an increase in TSH concentration up to $\geq$ 10 mU/l is observed, then permanent CH is confirmed. On the other hand, if the thyroid function remains normal, the dose can be reduced further. In transient cases, this leads to the complete suspension of therapy.

Depending on the hormonal data at the end of re-evaluation, it is possible to distinguish between [10]:

- permanent CH, with a serum concentration of TSH $\geq$ 10mU/L and normal or reduced fT4 levels according to the age. Thus, after withdrawal, patients affected by permanent CH restart the L-T4 substitutive life-long therapy;

- transient CH, with a serum concentration of TSH and fT4 in the normal range according to the age. These patients suspend treatment definitively;
- persistent hyperthyrotropinemia, with a serum concentration of TSH between 5 and 10mU/L and normal fT4 levels according to the age. There are still no guidelines defining the TSH cut-off after which it is recommended to restart L-T4 therapy in patients with persistent hyperthyrotropinemia alone. The choice in these cases thus depends on the pediatrician, in discussion with the family [42]. In any case, studies on this topic have not shown a significant benefit of L-T4 substitution in the outcome of these patients [43, 44], and thus it remains an open issue.

At the time of re-evaluation, the etiology of the thyroid dysfunction could be revealed. For this reason, a thyroid ultrasound is performed and, in selected cases, also a scintigraphy with ^{123}I, possibly followed by a perchlorate discharge test. The ultrasonography finding of a thyroid gland with a volume at the lower limit of the normal range may be due to the long-term substitutive therapy with L-T4 [10].

A normal or slightly reduced thyroid volume on ultrasound together with a low or absent tracer uptake on scintiscan, suggest the molecular analysis of the TSH-receptor gene, since in this situation resistance to TSH is possible [8]. The mutation of this gene in heterozygosity does not usually require life-long substitutive therapy, even though it causes persistent hyperthyrotropinemia.

If ultrasonography shows an eutopic thyroid gland with normal or increased volume and a greedy tracer uptake on scintiscan, this represents the characteristic pattern of dyshormonogenesis [8, 10]. This, combined with a high thyroglobulin serum level at diagnosis and a positive familial history of thyroid disease, raises the suspicion of an iodine organification defect, which should be investigated by a ^{123}I scintigraphy with a perchlorate discharge test [9]. This ion is a competitive inhibitor of the thyroid sodium-iodide symporter. Thus, interfering with iodine uptake, it causes the release of the iodine not incorporated into thyroglobulin into the bloodstream.

Therefore a reduction of ≥ 10% in the ^{123}I uptake levels at 2 hours after oral administration of sodium perchlorate is considered positive for an iodine organification defect (IOD). Patients with an iodine discharge of 10% to 90% are considered to have partial IOD and should then be investigated for *DUOX2* and *DUOXA2* mutations. On the other hand, patients with an iodine discharge greater than 90% are considered to have total IOD and should be evaluated for mutations in the thyroid peroxidase gene (*TPO*) [10].

Finally, the ultrasonographic finding of a normal or increased thyroid volume together with a high serum TSH and very low or non-detectable serum thyroglobulin, suggest a thyroglobulin synthesis defect. In these patients the molecular genetic analysis of the *thyroglobulin* gene should be carried out [9].

6. About Our Experience

In our program of neonatal screening in Emilia-Romagna (northern Italy, total inhabitants: 4.448.841) from January 2003 to December 2013, a total of 454.024 children were screened for CH, dosing TSH on dried blood spot (DBS) collected between 48 and 72 hours of life. The recall threshold was 12 mU/L up to 2007, then 10 mU/L to date. A total of 491 newborns were then recalled for an abnormal TSH value on DBS and the diagnosis of CH was confirmed in 405/491 (82.5%). Therefore the incidence of confirmed CH in Emilia- Romagna in this period was 1:1121 births. 280/405 infants showed a normally located gland, while the other 125 were found to have thyroid dysgenesis.

In patients with *in situ* gland we found a definitive diagnosis in 107/280 cases. Ninety-three of these patients underwent a re-evaluation of the diagnosis after the age of 3, while the others were considered to be affected by permanent CH due to the need to progressively increase the dosage of substitutive therapy during follow-up.

The re-evaluation was performed by decreasing the L-T4 dose by 30% for 2 to 3 weeks. If during this period an increase in TSH concentration up to ≥ 10mU/l was observed, then the diagnosis of permanent CH was confirmed. Otherwise, if the thyroid function remained normal, the dose was reduced further, leading to the complete suspension of therapy in transient cases. Depending on the hormonal data at the end of the re-evaluation, our patients were divided into three groups: 1) permanent CH, with a serum concentration of TSH ≥ 10 mU/L and normal or reduced fT4 levels according to the age; 2) transient CH, with a serum concentration of TSH and fT4 in the normal range according to the age; 3) persistent hyperthyrotropinemia, with a serum concentration of TSH between 5 and 10mU/L and normal fT4 levels according to the age.

Overall, of the 107 patients examined, the final diagnoses were:

- 28/107 (26%) permanent CH (14 after re-evaluation, the other 14 according to the trend of therapy during the follow-up);
- 31/107 (29%) persistent hyperthyrotropinemia;
- 48/107 (45%) transient CH.

Therefore 55% of patients were affected by a permanent thyroid dysfunction. Of these, a partial form of organification defect was detected in 34.5% of subjects submitted to the perchlorate test and TSH resistance due to a heterozygous mutation of the TSH-receptor gene was detected in 28.6%.

In the group with persistent hyperthyreotropinemia, 19/31 patients had to resume therapy due to an increasing trend of TSH > 10 mU/L during the follow-up, while the other 12 patients discontinued therapy but continued follow-up.

Almost half of the analyzed patients (45%) showed a complete normalization of the thyroid function after therapy withdrawal and, as previously mentioned, another 12% discontinued therapy despite a mild alteration in TSH.

In our cohort of patients, the prevalence of preterm infants (14.3%) was higher than that of the general population in Italy (5.2% in 2013 [45]). This means that prematurity may represent a risk factor for CH with *in situ* thyroid gland, in line with other data from the literature [11]. However, there were no significant differences in the incidence of preterm babies in the three groups of patients (permanent CH, transient CH, persistent hyperthyrotropinemia), thus prematurity cannot be used to predict the evolution of CH.

Analyzing various clinical and biochemical features at diagnosis and then at re-evaluation, we tried to reveal the possible predictive factors. The results showed that the mean dose of L-T4 taken by patients before starting re-evaluation was higher in the group affected by permanent thyroid dysfunction. This difference was more significant, from a statistical point of view, by comparing the group of infants who had to resume therapy with the group of infants who discontinued it. The mean dose of L-T4 could thus be used to predict the need for life-long therapy in this kind of patients.

Another difference concerns the thyroid volume on the ultrasound scan performed at the beginning of the re-evaluation. Patients affected by transient CH more often showed a thyroid of normal volume, compared with patients affected by permanent dysfunction.

Another interesting finding of our study regards the increase in the incidence of CH with *in situ* thyroid gland, as a result of the reduction in the recall threshold of TSH in the neonatal screening from 12 to 10 mU/L in 2007. Keeping this cut-off of 12 mU/L, we would have missed 42 diagnoses of CH in the neonatal age, 18 of whom were affected by permanent thyroid dysfunction.

CONCLUSION

In recent decades, there has been a progressive increase in the incidence of CH, especially with *in situ* thyroid gland. As emerged from our study and from many others in the literature, almost half of CH patients with *in situ* gland are in reality affected by a transient dysfunction, and therefore do not require life-long replacement therapy. This high percentage underlines the importance of the re-evaluation of the diagnosis in this group of patients, in order to avoid unnecessary therapies.

The frequent persistence of thyroid dysfunction in patients with borderline TSH values at the NS highlights the importance of reducing the recall threshold. A lower TSH recall threshold enables CH to be diagnosed in some patients that show a delayed increase in serum TSH, such as preterm babies [46], thus preventing false negative results. According to European guidelines, preterm and other special categories of newborns at risk for CH (LBW and VLBW neonates; ill and preterm neonates admitted to the NICU; twins, particularly in same sex cases) should follow a special screening procedure, based on multiple samplings: the first specimen is collected as usual at 48-72 hours of life, and then the second one, 2 weeks later [8].

REFERENCES

[1] Rastogi, MV; LaFranchi, SH. Congenital hypothyroidism. *Orphanet J Rare Dis*, 2010, 25(1-2), 13-29.

[2] Grüters, A; Krude, H. Detection and treatment of congenital hypothyroidism. *Nat Rev Endocrinol*, 2012, 8(2), 104-113.

[3] Fisher, DA. Second International Conference on Neonatal Thyroid Screening: Progress report. *J Pediatr*, 1983, 102, 653-654.

[4] Ford, G; Lafranchi, SH. Screening for congenital hypothyroidism: A worldwide view of strategies. *Best Pract Res Clin Endocrinol Metab*, 2014, 28(2), 175-187.

[5] Corbetta, C; Weber, G; Cortinovis, F; Calebiro, D; Passoni, A; Vigone, MC; Beck-Peccoz, P; Chiumello, G; Persani, L. A 7-year experience with low blood TSH cutoff levels for neonatal screening reveals an unsuspected frequency of congenital hypothyroidism (CH). *Clin Endocrinol (Oxf)*, 2009, 71(5), 739-745.

[6] Mengreli, C; Kanaka-Gantenbein, C; Girginoudis, P; Magiakou, MA; Christakopoulou, I; Giannoulia-Karantana, A; Chrousos, GP; Dacou-Voutetakis, C. Screening for congenital hypothyroidism:

The significance of threshold limit in falsenegative results. *J Clin Endocrinol Metab*, 2010, 95(9), 4283-4290.

[7] Wassner, AJ; Brown, RS. Congenital hypothyroidism. *Curr Opin Endocrinol Diabetes Obes*, 2015, 22(5), 407-412.

[8] Léger, J; Olivieri, A; Donaldson, M; Torresani, T; Krude, H;van Vliet, G; Polak, M; Butler, G. European society for paediatric endocrinology consensus guidelines on screening, diagnosis, and management of congenital hypothyroidism. *Horm Res Paediatr*, 2014, 81(2), 80-103.

[9] Cassio, A; Corbetta, C; Antonozzi, I; Calaciura, F; Caruso, U; Cesaretti, G; Gastaldi, R; Medda, E; Mosca, F; Pasquini, E; Salerno, MC; Stoppioni, V; Tonacchera, M; Weber, G; Olivieri, A. The Italian screening program for primary congenital hypothyroidism: Actions to improve screening, diagnosis, follow-up, and surveillance. *J Endocrinol Invest*, 2013, 36(3), 195-203.

[10] Rabbiosi, S; Vigone, MC; Cortinovis, F; Zamproni, I; Fugazzola, L; Persani, L; Corbetta, C; Chiumello, G; Weber, G. Congenital Hypothyroidism With Eutopic Thyroid Gland: Analysis of Clinical and Biochemical Features at Diagnosis and After Re-Evaluation. *J Clin Endocrinol Metab*, 2013, 98(4), 1395-1402.

[11] Olivieri, A; Fazzini, C; Medda, E. Multiple factors influencing the incidence of congenital hypothyroidism detected by neonatal screening. *Horm Res Paediatr*, 2015, 83(2), 86-93.

[12] Castanet, M; Polak, M; Bonaïti-Pellié, C; Lyonnet, S; Czernichow, P; Léger, J. Nineteen years of national screening for congenital hypothyroidism: familial cases with thyroid dysgenesis suggest the involvement of genetic factors. *J Clin Endocrinol Metab*, 2001, 86, 2009-2014.

[13] Bubuteishvili, L; Garel, C; Czernichow, P; Leger, J. Thyroid abnormalities by ultrasonography in neonates with congenital hypothyroidism. *J Pediatr*, 2003, 143, 759-764.

[14] Cassio, A; Bal, MO; Bettocchi, I; Baronio, F. Thyroid Enlargement from Newborn to Adolescent. In: G. Bona et al. *Thyroid Diseases in Childhood: Recent Advances from Basic Science to Clinical Practice*. Switzerland: Springer, 2015, 147-156.

[15] Al Taji, E; Biebermann, H; Límanová, Z; Hníková, O; Zikmund, J; Dame, C; Grüters, A; Lebl, J; Krude, H. Screening for mutations in transcription factors in a Czech cohort of 170 patients with congenital and early-onset hypothyroidism: identification of a novel PAX8 mutation in dominantly inherited early-onset non-autoimmune hypothyroidism. *Eur J Endocrinol*, 2007, 156, 521-529.

[16] Grasberger, H; Refetoff, S. Genetic causes of congenital hypothyroidism due to dyshormonogenesis. *Curr Opin Pediatr*, 2011, 23, 421-428.

[17] Biebermann, H; Schoneberg, T; Krude, H; Schultz, G; Gudermann, T; Grüters, A. Mutations of the human thyrotropin receptor gene causing thyroid hypoplasia and persistent congenital hypothyroidism. *J Clin Endocrinol Metab*, 1997, 82, 3471-3480.

[18] Grasberger, H; Mimouni-Bloch, A; Vantyghem, MC; van Vliet, G; Abramowicz, M; Metzger, DL; Abdullatif, H; Rydlewski, C; Macchia, PE; Scherberg, NH; van Sande, J; Mimouni, M; Weiss, RE; Vassart, G; Refetoff, S. Autosomal dominant resistance to thyrotropin as a distinct entity in five multigenerational kindreds: clinical characterization and exclusion of candidate loci. *J Clin Endocrinol Metab*, 2005, 90, 4025-4034.

[19] Olivieri, A; Radetti, G; Medda, E. Incidence of congenital hypothyroidism in the Autonomous Province of Bolzano: Benefit of increased iodine intake. *J Endocrinol Invest*, 2015, 38(2), 185-187.

[20] Huang, SA; Tu, HM; Harney, JW; Venihaki, M; Butte, AJ; Kozakewich, HPW; Fishman, SJ; Larsen, PR. Severe Hypothyroidism caused by type 3 Iodothyronine Deiodinase in Infantile Hemangiomas. *New England Journal of Medicine*, 2000, 343(3), 185-189.

[21] Weber, G; Rabbiosi, S; Zamproni, I; Fugazzola, L. Genetic defects of hydrogen peroxide generation in the thyroid gland. *J Endocrinol Invest*, 2013, 36(4), 261-266.

[22] Jin, HY; Heo, SH; Kim, YM; Kim, GH; Choi, JH; Lee, BH; Yoo, HW. High frequency of DUOX2 mutations in transient or permanent congenital hypothyroidism with eutopic thyroid glands. *Horm Res Paediatr*, 2014, 82(4), 252-260.

[23] Delange, F. Neonatal screening for congenital hypothyroidism: results and perspectives. *Horm Res*, 1997, 48, 51–61.

[24] Tylek-Lemańska, D; Rybakova, M; Kumorowicz-Kopiec, M; Dziatkowiak, H; Ratajczak, R. Iodine deficiency disorders incidence in neonates based on the experience with mass screening for congenital hypothyroidism in southeast Poland in the years 1985–2000. *J Endocrinol Invest*, 2003, 26, 32-38.

[25] Olivieri, A; Radetti, G; Medda, E. Incidence of congenital hypothyroidism in the Autonomous Province of Bolzano: benefit of increased iodine intake. *J Endocrinol Invest*, 2015, 38, 185-187.

[26] Olivieri, A; Corbetta, C; Weber, G; Vigone, MC; Fazzini, C; Medda, E. Congenital hypothyroidism due to defects of thyroid development and mild increase of TSH at screening: Data from the Italian National Registry of infants with congenital hypothyroidism. *J Clin Endocrinol Metab*, 2013, 98(4), 1403-1408.

[27] Belfort, MB; Pearce, EN; Braverman, LE; He, X; Brown, RS. Low iodine content in the diets of hospitalized preterm infants. *J Clin Endocrinol Metab*, 2012, 97(4), 632-636.

[28] Alm, J; Larsson, A; Zetterström, R. Congenital hypothyroidism in Sweden. Incidence and age at diagnosis. *Acta Paediatr Scand*, 1978, 67, 1-3.

[29] Alm, J; Hagenfeldt, L; Larsson, A; Lundberg, K. Incidence of congenital hypothyroidism: retrospective study of neonatal laboratory screening versus clinical symptoms as indicators leading to diagnosis. *Br Med J (Clin Res Ed)*, 1984, 289(6453), 1171-1175.

[30] Mitchell, ML; Hsu, HW; Sahai, I. The increased incidence of congenital hypothyroidism: Fact or fancy? *Clin Endocrinol (Oxf)*, 2011, 75(6), 806-810.

[31] Harris, KB; Pass, KA. Increase in congenital hypothyroidism in New York State and in the United States. *Mol Genet Metab*, 2007, 91(3), 268-277.

[32] Deladoey, J; Ruel, J; Giguere, Y; Van Vliet, G. Is the incidence of congenital hypothyroidism really increasing? A 20-year retrospective

population-based study in Quebec. *J Clin Endocrinol Metab*, 2011, 96(8), 2422-2429.

[33] Albert, BB; Cutfield, WS; Webster, D; Carll, J; Derraik, JG; Jefferies, C; Gunn, AJ; Hofman, PL. Etiology of increasing incidence of congenital hypothyroidism in New Zealand from 1993-2010. *J Clin Endocrinol Metab*, 2012, 97(9), 3155-3160.

[34] Kurinczuk, JJ; Bower, C; Lewis, B; Byrnee, G. Congenital hypothyroidism in Western Australia 1981-1998. *Journal of Pediatrics and Child Health*, 2002, 38, 187-191.

[35] Olivieri, A. The Study Group for Congenital Hypothyroidism. The Italian National Register of infants with congenital hypothyroidism: twenty years of surveillance and study of congenital hypothyroidism. *Ital J Pediatr*, 2009, 35, 2.

[36] Kempers, MJE; Lanting, CI; Van Heijst, AFJ; van Trotsenburg, AS; Wiedijk, BM; de Vijlder, JJ; Vulsma, T. Neonatal screening for congenital hypothyroidism based on thyroxine, thyrotropin, and thyroxinebinding globulin measurement: Potentials and pitfalls. *J Clin Endocrinol Metab*, 2006, 91(9), 3370-3376.

[37] Beck, S; Wojdyla, D; Say, L; Betran, AP; Merialdi, M; Harris Requejo, J; Rubens, C; Menon, R; Van Look, PFA. The worldwide incidence of preterm birth: A systematic review of maternal mortality and morbidity. *Bull World Health Organ*, 2010, 88(1), 31-38.

[38] Reynolds, MA; Schieve, LA; Martin, JA; Jeng, G; Macaluso, M. Trends in multiple births conceived using assisted reproductive technology, United States, 1997-2000. *Pediatrics*, 2003, 111(5 Part 2), 1159-1162.

[39] Collins, J. Global epidemiology of multiple birth. *Reprod Biomed Online*, 2007, 15, 45-52.

[40] Olivieri, A; Medda, E; De Angelis, S; Valensise, H; De Felice, M; Fazzini, C; Cascino, I; Cordeddu, V; Sorcini, M; Stazi, MA. Study Group for Congenital Hypothyroidism. High Risk of Congenital Hypothyroidism in Multiple Pregnancies. *J Clin Endocrinol Metab*, 2007, 92(8), 3141-3147.

[41] Hinton, CF; Harris, KB; Borgfeld, L; Drummond-Borg, M; Eaton, R;, Lorey, F; Therrell, BL; Wallace, J; Pass, KA. Trends in Incidence Rates of Congenital Hypothyroidism Related to Select Demographic Factors: Data From the United States, California, Massachusetts, New York, and Texas. *Pediatrics*, 2010, 125(Supplement), S37-S47.

[42] Castanet, M; Goischke, A; Léger, J; Thalassinos, C; Rodrigue, D; Cabrol, S; Zenaty, D; al-Harbi, M; Polak, M; Czernichow, P. Fédération Parisienne pour le Dépistage et la Prévention des Handicaps de l'Enfant (FDPHE). Natural history and management of congenital hypothyroidism with in situ thyroid gland. *Horm Res Paediatr*, 2015, 83(2), 102-110.

[43] O'Grady, MJ; Cody, D. Subclinical hypothyroidism in childhood. *Arch Dis Child*, 2011, 96(3), 280-284.

[44] Wasniewska, M; Corrias, A; Aversa, T; Valenzise, M; Mussa, A; De Martino, L; Lombardo, F; De Luca, F; Salerno, M. Comparative evaluation of therapy with l-thyroxine versus no treatment in children with idiopathic and mild subclinical hypothyroidism. *Horm Res Paediatr*, 2012, 77(6), 376-381.

[45] http://www.salute.gov.it/imgs/C_17_pubblicazioni_2431_allegato.pdf.

[46] Woo, HC; Lizarda, A; Tucker, R; Mitchell, ML; Vohr, B; Oh, W; Phornphutkul, C. Congenital hypothyroidism with a delayed thyroid-stimulating hormone elevation in very premature infants: Incidence and growth and developmental outcomes. *J Pediatr*, 2011, 158(4), 538-542.

In: Advances in Health and Disease. Volume 4 ISBN: 978-1-53613-345-5
Editor: Lowell T. Duncan

Chapter 7

BURKITT'S LYMPHOMA: ETIOLOY, PATHOLOGY, PROGNOSIS AND TREATMENT

Seema Naik*
Penn State Cancer Institute
Hershey, Pennsylvania, PA, US

ABSRACT

Etiology: There are three types of Burkitt's Lymphoma: Endemic (African), Sporadic (non-African) and HIV-associated per WHO classification. Compared to the endemic type which is commonly associated with EBV infection, the incidence of EBV is lower in the other two types (20% in sporadic and 30- 40% in HIV patients). Burkitt's Lymphoma is distinguished from diffuse large-B-cell lymphoma by the high level of expression of c-myc, the expression of germinal-center B-cell genes, and the low level of MHC class I genes and nuclear factor-kappa target genes.

* Corresponding Author Email: snaik@pennstatehealth.psu.edu.

Immunodeficiency-associated Burkitt's lymphoma occurs mainly in patients infected with HIV but also occurs in allograft recipients and individuals with congenital immunodeficiency. Burkitt's lymphoma accounts for 30%–40% of non-Hodgkin's lymphoma in HIV+ patients. Burkitt's lymphoma is estimated to be 1,000 times more common in HIV+ individuals. HIV+ patients with Burkitt's lymphoma are younger, less often carry a prior diagnosis of AIDS, and have higher mean CD4 counts. HIV-associated Burkitt's lymphoma shares some pathogenetic features with endemic Burkitt's lymphoma.

Patients with Burkitt's lymphoma have a median age of 54.5 years with a CR rate of 72% and a lymphoma free long-time survival of 55%. The International Prognostic Index IPI is the most valuable prognostic factor for survival. Favorable disease by Murphy's system is stage I or stage IIR and normal LDH.

Symptoms: Endemic Burkitt's lymphoma most commonly involves the maxilla and/or mandible; however, abdominal organs may also be involved. A tumor can double in size in 18 hours. Presentation is commonly with swelling of the affected jaw bones and rapidly enlarging, non-tender lymph nodes in the neck or jaw. Sporadic Burkitt's lymphoma usually involves the abdominal organs, most frequently the distal ileum, caecum or mesentery. Other abdominal and pelvic organs, glandular tissue (such as the thyroid and tonsils) and the facial bones may also be involved. Presentation is commonly with abdominal mass/swelling and ascites, intestinal obstruction. B symptoms may be present with both forms of Burkitt's lymphoma and include fever, weight loss, night sweats. HIV-related Burkitt's lymphoma tends to present in a similar way to the sporadic disease.

Treatment Options: Treatment of Burkitt's lymphoma in younger and fit patients is R-HyperCVAD, R-CODOX/MVAC. For low-risk disease with single site of disease <10 cm and a normal LDH, 3 cycles of R-CODOX-M are considered. For older patients more than 60 years of age R-EPOCH is preferred but R-HyperCVAD could be considered for select older fit patients.

Salvage chemotherapy options for relapsed Burkitt's lymphoma are aggressive CCE or other ALL induction regimens. Allogeneic transplants may be considered for fit patients who obtain second CR. The patient should receive CNS prophylaxis with each cycle of chemotherapy.

For HIV-related Burkitt's lymphoma, a dose-Adjusted R-EPOCH is again considered a preferred treatment. For young, fit patients with well-controlled HIV and good $CD4^+$ counts R-HyperCVAD and R-CODOX-M/IVAC could be considered as alternative treatment options. The overall survival is superior among those who receive intensive chemotherapy regimens instead of lower-dose regimens.

BACKGROUND

Burkitt's lymphoma (BL) is the most common form of non-Hodgkin lymphoma occurring in children and adolescents. Burkitt's is the most common in children in Africa with some evidence linking its etiology to Epstein-Barr virus [1]. In Africa, BL is common in young children who also have malaria and Epstein-Barr virus that causes infectious mononucleosis. One mechanism may be that malaria weakens the immune system's response to Epstein-Barr, allowing it to change infected B-cells into cancerous cells. About 98% of African cases are associated with EBV infection. Outside of Africa, BL is rare. In the U.S., about 1,200 people are diagnosed each year, and approximately 59% of patients are over age 40. Burkitt's lymphoma (BL) is especially likely to develop in HIV infected people with the incidence of BL estimated to be 1,000 times higher in HIV-positive people than in the general population before the HAART era.

Types of Burkitt's Lymphoma

In the World Health Organization (WHO) classification, there are three types of Burkitt's lymphoma:

1. Endemic (African): Endemic Burkitt's lymphoma primarily affects African children ages 4 to 7 and is twice as common in boys.
2. Sporadic (non-African): Sporadic Burkitt's lymphoma occurs worldwide. Globally, it accounts for 1% to 2% of adult lymphoma cases. In the U.S. and Western Europe, it accounts for up to 40% of pediatric lymphoma cases.
3. Immunodeficiency-associated: This variant of Burkitt's lymphoma is most common in people with HIV/AIDS. It accounts for 30% to 40% of non-Hodgkin lymphoma in HIV patients and may be an AIDS-defining disease. It also can occur in people with congenital

immune deficiency and in organ transplant patients on immunosuppressive drugs.

Compared to the endemic type, the incidence of EBV infection is considerably lower in the other two types of BL. In the sporadic disease, EBV is associated in about 20% of the patients. With the immunodeficiency-associated type, EBV is seen in 30-40% of patients. Association of EBV with these two types of BL is unclear.

EPIDEMIOLOGY

Dr. Denis Parsons Burkitt, MD, first studied and characterized the disease in equatorial Africa. It was during the medical mission to Uganda that he observed an increased frequency of children with masses in unusual sites including primarily in the jaw and neck. He proposed that BL was a type of malignancy [2]. Dr. Burkitt is credited for describing an endemic BL with a high incidence in equatorial Africa where it is the most common childhood cancer. The incidence of BL peaks between ages 4 and 7 years with an increased prevalence among males with nearly all cases EBV-seropositive. The sporadic form of BL also occurs primarily in children but maintains a predilection among males. The incidence in the US is around 0·6/100 000 per year among males and 0·2/100 000 among females aged 0–30 years. The classical sporadic presentation is associated with an abdominal mass, typically in the ileocecal region; however, lymph node, gonadal, and other organ involvement can be present at presentation. Most commonly, the sporadic form is associated with spread to the bone marrow and/or CNS at diagnosis with 30% EBV-positive case. Overall, BL has a trimodal pattern across with peaks at ages 10, 40, and 75 years among males. Recent increase in the incidence has been attributed to the increasing elderly population, secondary malignancy, and HIV-associated lymphoma [1, 2].

Histopathology

BL is a malignancy of mature B-cells of uniform, intermediate size with predominantly round nuclei. The nuclei show finely clumped chromatin with often multiple small, basophilic nucleoli. The cytoplasm is scant, basophilic, and demonstrates lipid vacuoles that are best appreciated on touch preparations or aspirate smears. The proliferation rate is extremely high with numerous mitotic figures and apoptotic bodies. These are engulfed in the cytoplasm of tingible body macrophages that are scattered throughout with characteristic 'starry sky' appearance from low power. Occasionally, increased nuclear pleomorphism and more prominent nucleoli are demonstrated.

Immunophenotype

BL cells express the B-cell antigens CD 19, CD 20, and CD 22 along with monotypic surface light chains. Consistent with their GCB origin, the cells express CD 10 and BCL 6. Nearly all cells (typically >99%) show expression of the proliferation antigen Ki-67, recognized by the antibody MIB-1. BCL 2 may be weakly positive in occasional cases, but strong positivity is not typical and should raise consideration of diagnosis of an indeterminate lymphoma [3].

Differential Diagnosis

Differential diagnostic considerations are typically limited to lymphoblastic leukemia/lymphoma, DLBCL, or the new entity in the 2008 WHO classification 'B-cell lymphoma, unclassifiable, with features intermediate between DLBCL and BL' (indeterminate B-cell lymphoma, IBL) [4]. The distinction between BL and lymphoblastic leukemia/

lymphoma is straightforward in most cases as the latter typically have finer chromatin, are CD 20 negative, and express TdT. However, in rare cases of lymphoblastic leukemia/lymphoma demonstrate mature features such as surface light chains and CD 20 expression. In these cases, cytogenetic analysis including karyotype and FISH for MYC rearrangement may be useful. DLBCL is usually distinguished from BL based on larger cell size with increased cytoplasm, greater nuclear pleomorphism, and lower Ki-67 proliferation index or strong BCL 2 staining. In DLBCL cases with less pleomorphism and a higher Ki-67, identification of a MYC-IgH translocation would favor BL, while either a BCL 2 or BCL 6 without a MYC translocation would indicate DLBCL. Some cases may fall into the new IBL category and demonstrate a 'double hit' with translocations of MYC and BCL 2 or, less commonly, BCL 6 [3].

CYTOGENETICS

BL is characterized by translocation of MYC at 8q24.21 with the immunoglobulin heavy chain locus in the most case a (IGH, 14q32.33) with rare translocations with the light chain genes for kappa (IGK, 2p11.2) and lambda (IGL, 22q11.2). Myc translocations result in constitutive expression of the MYC gene driven by the immunoglobulin gene enhancer. Recurrent chromosomal abnormalities d involving chromosomes 1, 6, 13, 17, and 22 have been recently recognized [5]. The main BL-associated chromosomal aberrations including + 1q (29%), +7q (14%), and del (13q) (14%) were also recently characterized in a large cytogenetic study. Either isolated 13q deletions or unbalanced translocations with 13q34 deletion were seen in 82% cases. The + 7q and del (13q) were independently associated with poor survival [6].

Gene Expression Profiling

Concurrent studies published in 2006 sought to define an expression profile signature of BL that would distinguish it from DLBCL. Dave et al. (2006) studied 45 BL cases and further divided into classic BL or atypical BL based on the 2001 WHO Classification, and compared them to 223 DLBCLs. The molecular classifier was developed based on genes differentially expressed between the BL and DLBCL as well as a set of MYC target genes. This molecular BL (mBL) signature included increased expression of MYC target genes, and GCB genes with decreased expression of MHC Class I genes and NF-κB target genes. All 25 cases of BL, and 19/20 cases of atypical BL, were classified as BL by the molecular classifier [7]. All cases diagnosed as DLBCL on pathology review were correctly classified. However, 31% of cases that were originally diagnosed as BL or atypical BL, but reclassified by pathology review as DLBCL, were classified as mBL by the algorithm suggesting that there is a subset of morphological DLBCL with an expression profile more consistent with BL. The cases with a pathological diagnosis of DLBCL and typical gene-expression profile of BL, suggest that these represent cases of Burkitt's lymphoma that are difficult to diagnose by current methods. Among 28 of the patients with a molecular diagnosis of BL, the overall survival was superior among those who had received intensive chemotherapy regimens instead of lower-dose regimens [8].

Risk Classification

At presentation, the majority of children and adolescents with non-Hodgkin lymphoma (NHL) present with advanced stage disease and/or metastasis. The original Murphy staging system [9] was adapted from that used for Hodgkin lymphoma (HL) and incorporates the metastatic nature of this illness based on the extent of nodal and/or extranodal involvement (Table 1). However, this staging system does not specifically address all subgroups of BL. The FAB and BFM staging based on the Murphy staging system further elucidate presentation characteristics specific to BL and DLBCL (Tables 2 and 3) [10].

Table 1. Murphy's staging system

Stage I	A single tumor (extranodal) or single anatomic area (nodal), with the exclusion of mediastinum or abdomen
Stage II	A single tumor (extranodal) with regional node involvement
	Two single (extranodal) tumors on the same side of the diaphragm with or without regional node involvement
	Primary gastrointestinal tract tumor with or without involvement of associated mesenteric nodes only
	Two or more nodal areas on the same side of the diaphragm
Stage IIR	Completely resected intra-abdominal disease
Stage III	Two single extranodal tumors on opposite sides of the diaphragm
	All primary intrathoracic tumors (mediastinal, pleural, thymic)
	All paraspinal or epidural tumors, regardless of other tumour sites
	All extensive primary intra-abdominal diseases
	Two or more nodal areas on opposite sides of the diaphragm
Stage IIIA	Localized but nonresectable intra-abdominal disease
Stage IIIB	Widespread multiorgan abdominal disease
Stage IV	Any of the above with initial central nervous system and/or bone marrow involvement (<25% involvement; >25% involvement is defined as L3/acute lymphocytic leukaemia

Table 2. BFM Burkitt's lymphoma risk classification

Risk	Resection	Stage	LDH (u/l)	CNS	
R1	Complete		I+II	Any	
R2	Incomplete		I+II	Any	
			III	<500	
R3			III	500–1000	
			IV, B-ALL	<1000	Negative
R4			III, IV, B-ALL	≥1000	
				Any	Positive

BFM, Berlin Frankfurt Munster; LDH, lactate dehydrogenase.
CNS, central nervous system; B-ALL, B-cell acute lymphocytic leukaemia.

Table 3. FAB Burkitt's Lymphoma Risk Stratification

FAB, French–American–British; CNS, central nervous system.
Group A
Completely resected Stage I
Completely resected abdominal Stage II lesions
Group B
All patients not eligible for Group A or Group C
Group C
Any CNS involvement and/or bone marrow involvement ≥25% blasts

Table 4. Comparison of BFM and FAB Classification

Berlin-Frankfurt-Munster (BFM)	French-American-British (FAB
R1 Stage I or II, completely resected	Group A Resected stage I and abdominal completely resected stage II
R2 Stage I or II, not resected Stage III with LDH <500 U/l	Group B
R3 Stage III with LDH >500 to 1000U/l Stage IV with LDH > 1000U/l and/or CNS negative	All patients not in Group A or Group C
R4 Stage III or Stage IV with LDH > 1000 U/l and/or CNS positive	Group C Bone Marrow disease (>25% L3 blasts) and/or CNS positive

Symptoms of Burkitt's Lymphoma

The symptoms of Burkitt's lymphoma depend on the type. The endemic (African) variant usually presents with tumors of the jaw or facial bones. It also can affect the gastrointestinal tract, ovaries, and breasts and can spread to the central nervous system, causing damage, weakness, and paralysis. The sporadic and immunodeficiency-associated types are more commonly seen in the U.S. and usually start in the bowel presenting with bulky tumor mass in the abdomen, often with common involvement of the liver, spleen, and bone marrow. These variants also can involve the ovaries, testes, or other organs, and spread to the brain and spinal fluid. Burkitt's lymphoma patients may also present with B symptoms including the loss of appetite, weight, Fatigue, Night sweats, unexplained fever.

Diagnosis of Burkitt's Lymphoma

Because Burkitt's lymphoma spreads so quickly, prompt diagnosis is essential. Once Burkitt's lymphoma is suspected, biopsy of an enlarged lymph node or other suspicious disease site is essential to confirm the diagnosis of Burkitt's lymphoma. Additional tests may include: Computed tomographic (CT) imaging of the chest, abdomen, and pelvis, chest X-ray, PET scan, Examination of spinal fluid, Blood tests to measure kidney and liver function, Testing for HIV disease.

Variants

HIV Associated Burkitt's Lymphoma

Endemicity is pathogenetically linked to an imbalance of the immune system which occurs in African children infected by malaria parasites and Epstein-Barr virus, while the epidemic form of BL strictly follows the pattern of infection by HIV. Highly active antiretroviral therapy (HAART) has extended the life expectancy of HIV/AIDS patients to approach that of the general population. However, it remains unclear whether HIV infection affects the survival of lymphoma patients in the HAART era. Among, the 179,520 lymphoma patients identified from the National Cancer Database during 2004-2011, the prevalence of HIV-infection ranged from 1.0% for FL, 3.3% for PTCL, 4.7 for HL, 5.4% for DLBCL, to 29% for BL. HIV infection was significantly associated with inferior overall survival for patients with each lymphoma subtype. (HR for Burkitt's lymphoma 1.46) (CI 1.24-1.73). HIV is independently associated with increased risk of death among lymphoma patients in the HAART era in the U.S. Consideration of effective management strategies for patients with HIV/AIDS-associated lymphoma and enrolment of patients in prospective clinical trials are needed to improve patient outcomes [11]. One of the challenges of most standard approaches typically used is severe treatment-related toxicity that often leads to discontinuation of therapy especially in the HIV infected population. There has been recent success developing intermediate intensity approaches such as dose adjusted R-EPOCH in this setting which are well tolerated in this patient group and maintain high cure rates [12].

Burkitt's Lymphoma Presenting Like PTLD

A variety of lymphomas can develop as PTLD, although some types appear infrequently and remain poorly understood. PTLD-Burkitt's lymphomas behave aggressively and require intensive chemotherapeutic intervention. The tumors display the typical histological features of Burkitt's lymphoma and are markedly positive for EBV [13]. Weak BCL2 expression is still compatible with the diagnosis of Burkitt's lymphoma. Contrary to common belief, strong BCL2 IHC expression is possible in typical Burkitt's lymphoma in adults and cannot be absolutely relied upon to distinguish between Burkitt's lymphoma and DLBCL [13]. Furthermore, the combination of a strong expression of BCL2 and EBV-positive status of the tumor suggests the disruption of an apoptotic pathway by EBV, promoting survival signals of the infected B cells [13, 14]. While BL-PTLD is a rare entity, it is a discrete form of PTLD, with a high EBV expression, and should be treated as a high-grade lymphoma. BL-PTLD historically represents a small, but significant, proportion of PTLD cases. BL-PTLD represents 15% of PTLD patients for pediatric heart, lung, and heart-lung transplants from 1982 to 2009, with a 1.1% overall incidence among pediatric transplant heart-lung recipients; 14% of our pediatric renal PTLD patients, 1.6% among kidney recipients; and 0.71% pediatric liver-transplant recipients, at a single institution study. BL-PTLD is a more aggressive type of PTLD and does not respond to a trial of decreased immunosuppression like P-PTLD and some M-PTLDs. BL-PTLD does require cessation of conventional immunosuppression during treatment with multiagent lymphoma-specific chemotherapy. Bone marrow involvement in the post-transplant setting remains a poor prognostic factor, despite of lymphoma-specific chemotherapy [15].

Burkitt's Like Lymphoma

Grey zone lymphomas are lymphomas that cannot be assigned to a defined lymphoma entity due to morphological, clinical or genetic reasons with features of two overlapping entities or features that are intermediate. The B-cell lymphoma, unclassified, with features intermediate between diffuse large B-cell lymphoma and Burkitt's lymphoma has recently been recognized as a provisional category in the updated WHO 2008 classification of malignant lymphomas. This corresponds to entities with a Burkitt's-like appearance and aggressive clinical behavior and are characterized by an atypical MYC translocation and complex karyotypic alterations [16]. The cases with a pathological diagnosis of diffuse large-B-cell lymphoma and typical gene-expression profile of Burkitt's lymphoma represent BL cases that are difficult to diagnose by current methods. For these patients with a molecular diagnosis of Burkitt's lymphoma, intensive chemotherapy regimens offer better survival outcomes [17].

PROGNOSIS

The overall survival is superior among those who receive intensive chemotherapy regimens instead of lower-dose regimens. Patients with BL with a median age of 54.5 years have a complete remission (CR) rate of 72% and a lymphoma free long-time survival of 55%. The International Prognostic Index IPI is the most valuable prognostic factor for survival. Favorable disease by Murphy's system [9] is stage I or stage IIR and normal LDH. Bone marrow involvement >25% is defined as L3 ALL and is not included in the staging system [10].

TREATMENTS FOR BURKITT'S LYMPHOMA

Intensive intravenous chemotherapy is the preferred treatment for Burkitt's lymphoma. Three decades ago, the prognosis of advanced (disseminated) BL in children and adolescents had a 5-year event free survival (EFS) of less than 40%, and required combination chemotherapy and radiation therapy over a 1–2 year period. Currently, the prognosis for the advanced stage has a 5-year EFS of 85–90% with less than 6 months of chemotherapy only. Radiation therapy has been eliminated for children and adolescents with BL except in emergencies, such as SVC syndrome and acute neurological impairment or in patients with relapse/progression. Current risk factors in the prognosis of childhood and adolescent BL include: LDH $\geq 2\times$ the upper normal limit at diagnosis, bone marrow and central nervous system involvement, poor response to cyclophosphamide, vincristine and prednisone reduction therapy and poor risk cytogenetics [18]. Since BL can spread to brain and CSF, intrathecal chemotherapy is important. The drugs used in various combinations for Burkitt's lymphoma include: cyclophosphamide, cytarabine, doxorubicin, etoposide, methotrexate, vincristine. CODOX M-IVAC is the most widely used regimen in adult Burkitt's lymphoma after the results of United Kingdom Lymphoma Group LY06 study [19]. In the late 1980s, Magrath and colleagues developed CODOX M/IVAC since more than half of children and adults treated with CHOP with methotrexate experienced disease recurrence [19]. In a subsequent study, investigators reduced the dose of methotrexate to 3 gm/m2 for patients younger than 65 years of age and 1 gm/m2 for patients older than 65 years of age and also reduced the dose of cytarabine in older patients to 1 gm/me. Fifty-three patients with a median age of 37 years were treated. The 2-year progression free survival (PFS) for all patients was 55% and was 85% and 49% for low- and high-risk patients, respectively.

Other treatments for BL may include intensive chemotherapy in combination with Rituximab, autologous stem cell transplantation, Radiation therapy and steroid therapy. In some cases, surgery may be needed for complications such as gastrointestinal bleeding, obstruction or rupture.

TREATMENT

Over the past three decades, the BFM regimens utilized a response-based therapy with variable doses of MTX [20]. They also added intensification phase with high dose cytarabine and etoposide for incomplete responders. These regimens including intraventricular chemotherapy, HD-MTX, were used to adequately treat CNS disease without irradiation. The BFM-95 study compared 24 hour continuous infusion HD-MTX and showed significant improvement for patients with CNS involvement [21]. Children's cancer group (CCG) evaluated treatment regimens, LSA2L2 or COMP in CCG-551 study with an improved outcome with COMP with a DFS 50% in children with nonlymphoblastic etiology. The subsequent CCG-5911 study investigated LMB 86 and a hybrid CCG regimen, which is a CHOP -like regimen followed an ifosfamide and etoposide followed by DECAL regimen with 2-year EFS 77% in CCG hybrid group with decrease in toxicity compared to LMB 86 [21].

Lymphoma malignancy B (LMB) group in their pilot study identified CNS disease as a significant risk factor. The LMB 84 study investigated a compressed chemotherapy regimen for patients without CNS involvement with 3-year EFS of 78% [22]. The LMB 89 study was able to demonstrate improvement in outcome for CNS positive patients similar to patient without CNS disease [23]. LMB 89 used a COPADM backbone with methotrexate at 3 g/m^2 for patients with Group B disease and 8 g/m^2 in patients with group C disease and the addition of high dose cytarabine and etoposide to Group C therapy. These regimens were associated with excellent outcomes in both intermediate risk (Group B) and advanced risk (Group C) with EFS of 94% and 85%, respectively. However, substantial toxicity including febrile neutropenia, mucositis, and systemic infections were seen [23].

Similarly, the Cancer and Leukemia Group B (CALGB) developed a regimen consisting of a prephase of cyclophosphamide and prednisone, followed by 3 cycles each of ifosfamide, methotrexate, vincristine, cytarabine, etoposide, dexamethasone alternating with cyclophosphamide, methotrexate, vincristine, doxorubicin, and dexamethasone [24]. Initially, patients received 2400 cGy of cranial irradiation and 12 doses of IT chemotherapy. The 5-year OS in 92 patients was 52%. In a follow-up study, 105 patients were treated with the addition of Rituximab in cycles 2 to 7. The 2-year EFS and OS were 74% and 78%, respectively. With the objective of evaluation of intensive chemotherapy with and without cranial radiation for central nervous system (CNS) prophylaxis in adults with Burkitt's leukemia or lymphoma, 18 weeks of therapy with prophylactic cranial radiation (2400 centigrays) and 12 doses of triple intrathecal chemotherapy were administered to the first cohort of patients. A subsequent cohort received intrathecal therapy for six doses and radiotherapy only to high-risk individuals. With the median follow-up of 6.8 years similar responses were seen with 3-year EFS 0.52 (95% CI, 0.38–0.65) and 0.45 (0.29–0.60). Intensive, short-duration chemotherapy with less intensive CNS prophylaxis led to control at this sanctuary site with little neurotoxicity and may be curative for adults with Burkitt's leukemia or lymphoma [25].

The group at MD Anderson developed HyperCVAD to treat acute lymphoblastic leukemia (ALL) and BL. Patients receive 4 cycles each of hyperfractionated cyclophosphosphamide with doxorubicin, vincristine, and dexamethasone alternating with 4 cycles of metotrexate and high-dose cytarabine. In their initial study of 26 adults, 5 patients died during induction. The 3-year OS was 49% and was 77% and 17% for patients under and over 60 years of age, respectively. In a subsequent prospective study of 31 patients treated with Rituximab plus HyperCVAD, the 3-year OS was significantly improved at 89%. Seventy-three percent of patients completed all therapy and severe myelosuppression was universal [26].

Ultimately, in an international collaborative study between CCG/COG, LMB, and (UKCCSG) in 1996, the patients with Group B or C disease were randomized to either standard LMB therapy or a dose-reduced regimen. Intermediate-risk Group B disease patients received 13 weeks of therapy with a deletion of maintenance COPADM3 and a 50% cyclophosphamide dose in COPADM2, with >90% 3-year EFS, and 2-year EFS 90% among Group C. Among Group C patients, bone marrow, CNS disease and poor COP reduction response were poor prognostic indicators [27]. Additional poor risk factors included primary mediastinal mass or presence of abdominal/retroperitoneal disease and LDH level ≥ two times upper normal limits

Recently, dose-adjusted EPOCH (etoposide, prednisone, vincristine, cyclophosphamide, adraimycin) plus Rituximab (DA-REPOCH) an infusional regimen designed to preserve efficacy while reducing toxicity was studies by Dunleavy and colleagues [12]. CNS prophylaxis consists of 8 doses of IT methotrexate with additional doses for patients with leptomeningeal involvement. With a median follow-up of more than 6 years, the DA-REPOCH patients achieved a freedom from progression of 95% and OS of 100%. The failure-free survival (FFS) and OS in the SC-EPOCH-RR (short-course R-EPOCH with a double dose of Rituximab) patients were 100% and 90%, respectively [12].

COMMON CHEMOTHERAPY BACKBONES

For older patients (>50), treatment with lymphoma protocols may yield response rates that are comparable to the results of patients with disseminated diffuse large cell lymphoma [12]. Younger patients with risk factors are treated with more intensive therapy like ALL-protocols. The role of autologous transplantation after high dose therapy (HDT) as part of primary treatment still needs to be evaluated in clinical trials. A common treatment paradigm for BL in children and adolescents is aimed at reduced toxicity while maintaining survival. The current chemotherapy backbones allow for the omission of cranial irradiation with a goal to reduce toxicity. Also, the use of methotrexate, doxorubicin and cyclophosphamide as mainstays of therapy is also clear among the FAB and BFM groups although no exact consensus exists on dosing and the use of additional chemotherapeutic agents. The role of autologous transplantation after high dose therapy (HDT) as part of primary treatment still needs to be evaluated in clinical trials.

Salvage Chemotherapy Options

Salvage chemotherapy options for relapsed Burkitt's lymphoma are aggressive CCE or other ALL induction regimens. Allogeneic transplants may be considered for fit patients who obtain second CR. The patient should receive CNS prophylaxis with each cycle of chemotherapy.

Tumor Lysis Syndrome (TLS)

Rapidly growing or bulky tumors with rapid doubling time can lead to tumor lysis resulting in hyperuricemia, hyperkalemia, hyperphosphatemia, hypocalcemia with or without renal failure. In the past, children with BL who received allopurinol prophylaxis had a 21% incidence of TLS requiring hemodialysis during induction chemotherapy. Aggressive medical management including laboratory monitoring, aggressive hydration, and use of allopurinol or a recombinant urate oxidase, rasburicase, to decrease and prevent hyperuricemia are required to prevent such complications. Goldman et al. demonstrated that rasburicase more rapidly lowers uric acid levels compared to allopurinol in children and adolescents at high risk of TLS [28, 29].

Immunotherapy

Rituximab has been used for the treatment of adults with CD20 positive B-cell lymphoma and recently also in children and adolescents with BL. One of the earlier studies investigating the use of Rituximab in this patient population observed the response of children with relapsed or refractory disease with 64% of patients with BL had a complete or partial response [30, 31]. Preliminary results of a large randomized study in 257 adults comparing the LMB regimen with and without Rituximab demonstrated significant improvement in 3-year EFS and OS in the Rituximab containing arms at 76% compared to 64% and 82% compared to 71%, respectively. In comparing the 2 HyperCVAD trials, the outcome in the Rituximab-containing study was clearly superior. Meinhardt et al. investigated the upfront usage of Rituximab in children with newly diagnosed mature B cell NHL and Burkitt's leukemia with 42% response rate to single agent Rituximab [32]. Cairo et al. also reported that Rituximab was safe and well-tolerated when combined with FAB B4 therapy in children with stage III/IV BL resulting in a 95% 3 year EFS [27]. Also, the addition of Rituximab to FAB Group C therapy for children and adolescents with CNS disease was associated with a 93% 3-year EFS and OS [30].

Future Directions

Because of its rarity and high curability, progress in advancing therapeutics in Burkitt's lymphoma (BL) has been difficult. Over recent years, several new mutations that cooperate with MYC have been identified, and this has paved the way for testing novel agents in the disease. New and novel therapeutic approaches include monoclonal antibody (anti-CD 20) therapy, targeted cellular immune therapy and small molecule inhibitors. Future strategies should include improved staging and risk classification, reduction of cytotoxic chemotherapy, the investigation of targeted therapy, an increased understanding of the underlying biology of Burkett's lymphoma/leukemia, strategies for prevention and approaches to reduce acute and chronic toxicities.

References

[1] Hochberg J, Waxman IM, Kelly KM, et al. Adolescent non-Hodgkin lymphoma and Hodgkin lymphoma: state of the science. *Br J Haematol.* 2009 Jan;144(1):24-40.

[2] Magrath IT. African Burkitt's lymphoma. History, biology, clinical features, and treatment. *Am J Pediatr Hematol Oncol.* 1991 Summer; 13(2):222-46. Review,

[3] Picarsic J, Jaffe R, Mazariegos G, Webber SA, Ellis D, Green MD, et al. Post-transplant Burkitt's lymphoma is a more aggressive and distinct form of post-transplant lymphoproliferative disorder. *Cancer.* 2011; 117:4540–4550.

[4] Campo E, Swerdlow SH, Harris NL, Pileri S, Stein H, Jaffe ES. The 2008 WHO classification of lymphoid neoplasms and beyond: evolving concepts and practical applications. *Blood.* 2011; 117(19):5019-32.

[5] Hummel M, Bentink S, Berger H, et al. A biologic definition of Burkitt's lymphoma from transcriptional and genomic profiling. *N Engl J Med.* 2006 Jun 8;354(23):2419-30.

[6] Poirel HA, Cairo MS, Heerema NA, et al. FAB/LMB 96 International Study Committee. Specific cytogenetic abnormalities are associated with a significantly inferior outcome in children and adolescents with mature B-cell non-Hodgkin's lymphoma: results of the FAB/LMB 96 international study. *Leukemia.* 2009.

[7] Dave SS, Fu K, Wright GW, Lam L, et al. Molecular diagnosis of Burkitt's lymphoma. Lymphoma/Leukemia Molecular Profiling Project. *N Engl J Med.* 2006 Jun 8; 354(23):2431-42.

[8] Bishop PC, Rao VK, Wilson WH. Burkitt's lymphoma: Molecular pathogenesis and treatment. *Cancer Invest* 2000; 18:574-83.

[9] Murphy SB. Classification, staging and end results of treatment of childhood non-Hodgkin's lymphomas: dissimilarities from lymphomas in adults. *Semin Oncol.* 1980 Sep; 7(3):332-9.

[10] Sandlund JT. Burkitt lymphoma: staging and response evaluation. *Br J Haematol*. 2012 Mar; 156(6):761-5.

[11] Han X, Jemal A, Hulland E, et al. HIV infection and survival of lymphoma patients in the era of highly active antiretroviral therapy. *Cancer Epidemiol Biomarkers Prev*. 2016.

[12] Dunleavy K, Little RF, Wilson WH· Update on Burkitt's lymphoma. *Hematol Oncol Clin North Am*. 2016 Dec; 30(6):1333-1343.

[13] Pervez S, Raza MQ, Mirza A, Pal A. Strong BCL2 expression in Burkitt's lymphoma is not uncommon in adults. *Indian J Pathol Microbiol.* 2011; 54:290–293.

[14] Kramer MH, Hermans J, Wijburg E, et al. Clinical relevance of BCL2, BCL6, and MYC rearrangements in diffuse large B-cell lymphoma. *Blood* 1998; 92:3152-62.

[15] Ott MM, Horn H, Rosenwald A, et al. Grey zone lymphomas: limitations of the classification of aggressive B-cell lymphomas. *Pathologe.* 2013 May; 34(3):225-32. (abstract).

[16] Butler RD, Hainsworth JD. Optimal therapy for small noncleaved cell lymphoma. *Cancer Treat Res* 1993; 66:65-79.

[17] Cairo M, Sposto R, Gerrard M, et al. Advanced Stage, Increased Lactate Dehydrogenase, and Primary Site, but Not Adolescent Age (≥ 15 Years), Are Associated With an Increased Risk of Treatment Failure in Children and Adolescents With Mature B-Cell Non-Hodgkin's Lymphoma: Results of the FAB LMB 96 Study. *J Clin Oncol*. 2012 Feb 1; 30(4): 387–393.

[18] Patte C, Auperin A, Gerrard M, et al. Results of the randomized international FAB/ LMB96 trial for intermediate risk B-cell non-

Hodgkin lymphoma in children and adolescents: it is possible to reduce treatment for the early responding patients. *Blood.* 2007 Apr 1; 109(7):2773-80.

[19] Mead GM, Sydes MR, Walewski J, et al. An international evaluation of CODOXM and CODOX-M alternating with IVAC in adult Burkitt's lymphoma: results of United Kingdom Lymphoma Group LY06 study. *Ann Oncol* 2002; 13:1264-74.

[20] Pees HW, Radtke H, Schwamborn J, Graf N. The BFM-protocol for HIV-negative Burkitt's lymphomas and L3 ALL in adult patients: a high chance for cure. *Ann Hematol* 1992; 65:201-5.

[21] Woessmann W, Seidemann K, Mann Getal; BFM Group. The impact of the methotrexate administration schedule and dose in the treatment of children and adolescents with B-cell neoplasms: a report of the BFM Group Study NHL-BFM95. *Blood.* 2005 Feb 1; 105(3):948-58.

[22] Philip T, Meckenstock R, Deconnick E, et al. Treatment of poor prognosis Burkitt's lymphoma in adults with the Société Française d'Oncologie Pédiatrique LMB Protocol--a study of the Federation Nationale des Centres de Lutte Contre le Cancer (FNLCC). *Eur J Cancer.* 1992; 28A (12):1954-9.

[23] Jourdain A, Auperin A, Minard-ColinV et al. Outcome of and prognostic factors for relapse in children and adolescents with mature B-cell lymphoma and leukemia treated in three consecutive prospective "*Lymphomes Malins B*" protocols. *A Société Française des Cancers de l'Enfant study Haematologica.* 2015 Jun; 100(6): 810–817.

[24] Larson RA, Dodge RK, Burns CP, et al. A five-drug remission induction regimen with intensive consolidation for adults with acute lymphoblastic leukemia: Cancer and Leukemia Group B study 8811. *Blood.* 1995; 85: 2025–2037.

[25] Rizzieri DA, Johnson JL, Niedzwiecki D, et al. Intensive chemotherapy with and without cranial radiation for Burkitt's leukemia and lymphoma: final results of Cancer and Leukemia Group B Study 9251. *Cancer* 2004;100(7):1438-1448.

[26] Thomas DA, Cortes J, O'Brien S, et al. Hyper-CVAD program in Burkitt's-type adult acute lymphoblastic leukemia. *J Clin Oncol* 1999;17:2461-70. 1. 2. 3. 4. 5. 6. 7.

[27] Cairo M, Gerrard M, Sposto R, et al. Results of a randomized international study of high-risk central nervous system B non-Hodgkin lymphoma and B acute lymphoblastic leukemia in children and adolescents. *Blood* 2007 109(7): 2736–2743.

[28] Cairo M, Sposto R, Gerrard M, et al. Advanced Stage, Increased Lactate Dehydrogenase, and Primary Site, but Not Adolescent Age (≥ 15 Years), Are Associated With an Increased Risk of Treatment Failure in Children and Adolescents With Mature B-Cell Non-Hodgkin's Lymphoma: Results of the FAB LMB 96 Study. *J Clin Oncol.* 2012 Feb 1; 30(4): 387–393.

[29] Cammalleri L,Malaguarnera M. Rasburicase represents a new tool for hyperuricemia in tumor lysis syndrome and in gout. *Int J Med Sci.* 2007; 4(2): 83–93.

[30] Goldman S, Smith L, Galardy P, et al. Rituximab with chemotherapy in children and adolescents with central nervous system and/or bone marrow-positive Burkitt's lymphoma/leukaemia: A Children's Oncology Group Report. *Br J Haematol.* 2014 Nov; 167(3): 394–401.

[31] Barnes JA, Lacasce AS, Feng Y, et al. Evaluation of the addition of Rituximab to CODOX-M/IVAC for Burkitt's lymphoma: a retrospective analysis. *Ann Oncol.* Vol. 22(8)2011.p.1859-1864.

[32] Griffin TC, Weitzman S, Weinstein H, et al. A Study of Rituximab and Ifosfamide, Carboplatin, and Etoposide Chemotherapy in Children with Recurrent/Refractory B-cell ($CD20^+$) Non-Hodgkin Lymphoma and Mature B-Cell Acute Lymphoblastic Leukemia: A Report from the Children's Oncology Group. *Pediatr Blood Cancer.* 2009 Feb; 52(2): 177–181.

In: Advances in Health and Disease. Volume 4 ISBN: 978-1-53613-345-5
Editor: Lowell T. Duncan

Chapter 8

CHALLENGES OF BLOOD PRESSURE MANAGEMENT IN PATIENTS WITH END-STAGE RENAL DISEASE

Shan Shan Chen, MD and Zhi Qiang Xu, MD
Nephrology Division, Department of Medicine at
the University of New Mexico School of Medicine,
Albuquerque, NM, US

ABSTRACT

Extremes of blood pressure are not uncommon in end stage renal disease (ESRD) patients that are associated with increased morbidities and mortalities. We will review the diagnosis, management and consequences of these in this chapter.

Interdialytic ambulatory blood pressure (ABP) or home BP, especially after the mid-week dialysis including the weekend, is the gold standard in diagnosis of hypertension in dialysis patients. Interdialytic ASBP of >130 mmHg or home SBP of >140 mmHg is associated with poor outcomes including mortality. Lowering of elevated BP in dialysis patients has shown to be beneficial. Treatment includes non-pharmacological measures, such as enhanced sodium removal with dialysis, dietary sodium restriction, probing of dry weight, prolonged dialysis duration and intensive dialysis treatment, and pharmacological measures. Selection of antihypertensive medications should take into consideration of underlying co-morbidities of the individuals, side effect profiles, and intra-and inter-dialytic pharmacokinetics of the medications. Beta-blocker is the preferred drug class among ESRD population due to its cardiovascular benefits. Low dialyzable beta-blockers are shown to have better mortality benefits than highly dialyzable ones. Calcium channel blockers, Angiotensin converting enzyme inhibitors and Angiotensin receptor blockers are also effective antihypertensive agents. Centrally acting alpha-agonist, direct vasodilators, and alpha-adrenergic blockers are adjunctive agents that are generally recommended for multidrug-resistant hypertension due to unfavorable side-effects and adherence concerns. Usage of mineralocorticoid receptor antagonists as antihypertensive agent is limited due to risk of hyperkalemia, but it is shown to minimize cardiovascular events in some studies. More data will be available after the completion of ALCHEMIST and SPin-D trials.

At the other end of the blood pressure spectrum, hypotension during or immediately following dialysis is an equally common phenomenon. Intradialytic hypotension (IDH) is defined by KDOQI guidelines as "a decrease systolic blood pressure by ≥20 mm Hg or a decrease in MAP by 10 mm Hg associated with symptoms." IDH carries a host of complications, including dysrhythmias, cardiac and cerebral ischemia, and fluid overload related to difficult ultrafiltration. It has been well known that there is "U"-shaped curve relationship between post-dialysis SBP and CV mortality in ESRD patients.

The risk factors for IDH include extremes of age, diabetics, cardiac dysfunction, coronary heart disease, and large interdialytic weight gains. Although IDH may occur due to serious underlying medical conditions, often no such causes are identified. The acute management of IDH consists of immediate reduction or discontinuation of ultrafiltration, administration of fluid bolus and oxygen, Trendelenburg position to increase cerebral perfusion. Long term conservative management of IDH encompasses reassessment of estimated dry weight, withholding antihypertensives before dialysis treatment, avoiding food intake just before and during dialysis, avoidance of large intradialytic weight gain, cool-temperature dialysate, use of midodrine, longer dialysis duration to allow for gentler ultrafiltration. In addition to these conservative measures, patients with persistent IDH will need a cardiac evaluation, including an echocardiogram.

INTRODUCTION

Extremes of blood pressures during dialysis are not uncommon and associated with increased morbidity and mortality in patients with end-stage renal disease (ESRD) [1, 2]. However, as their blood pressure (BP) values vary with timing and situation, treatment has become a challenge. This chapter will review the diagnosis, management and consequences of extreme BP in dialysis patient population.

HYPERTENSION

Diagnosis of Hypertension

For the general population, hypertension is defined as systolic blood pressure (SBP)/diastolic blood pressure (DBP) of ≥ 140/90 mmHg on the mean of 2 or more properly measured seated BP readings on each of two or more office visits [1]. However, it is unclear if this definition is applicable to the diagnosis of hypertension in patients with ESRD.

As BP values differ with different situations and timing in this unique population, it is a challenge to determine 1) which BP reading and 2) what BP value should be used for diagnosis of hypertension. Even with standardized BP measurement techniques, peri-dialysis BP values are not always representative of BP readings outside of the dialysis settings (interdialytic ambulatory BP (ABP) or home BP). It was found that pre-dialysis BP overestimated the ABP whereas post-dialysis BP underestimated the ABP [3].

Of the BP measurement techniques, ABP and home BP readings are preferred over peri-dialysis BP measurements in the diagnosis and treatment of hypertension due to their better correlation with target organ damage [4, 5]. Individuals with ESRD are considered to have hypertension when their interdialytic ASBP >130 mmHg or home SBP of >140 mmHg as BP values above these thresholds were associated with poor outcomes [6].

Even though outside-the-dialysis unit BP measurement is the gold standard, practically, it is challenging to obtain ABP or home BP. Dialysis unit BP measurements are easier to obtain. By using pre-dialysis BP values of 150/85 and 160/90 mmHg, it can reach at least 80% of sensitivity and specificity in the diagnosis of hypertension, respectively. A post-dialysis BP values of 130/75 and 140/80 will provide similar sensitivity and specificity, respectively [1].

Management of Hypertension

Blood Pressure Goal

KDOQI guideline from more than a decade ago recommended pre-dialysis and post-dialysis BP goals of <140/90 mmHg and <130/80 mmHg, respectively [7]. However, the recommendation was based on weak evidence and expert opinion. Previously, a "Reverse" or "U" curve relationship was noted between peri-dialysis BP and mortality. Normal or low BP was related to poor outcomes and high BP was found to have survival advantage. However, these were observational studies and the data for co-morbid conditions was lacking [8, 9]. The underlying illnesses, such as cardiac diseases and diabetes in elderly age population, and their severity can be a confounding factor in the reverse association between BP and mortality [10].

The positive association between higher peri-dialysis BP and mortality begs the question whether hypertension in dialysis patients should be treated and to what target. Meta-analysis of randomized controlled trials have shown cardiovascular benefits in lowering BP with antihypertensive medications [11].

Unlike the "U" curve relationship observed with peri-dialysis BP, ASBP and home SBP had linear correlation with mortality (hazard ratio, 1.26 [95% confidence interval, 1.14–1.40] per every 10 mmHg increase) [12]. Elevated outside-dialysis-unit SBP was associated with higher mortality and treatment of hypertension maybe beneficial to improve mortality.

However, there is no strong evidence what should be the SBP goal for dialysis patient population [9]. The Blood Pressure in Dialysis (BID) pilot study aimed to explore the safety and feasibility of performing randomized trial in dialysis patients to evaluate two SBP targets of 110 to 140 mm Hg or 155 to 165 mm Hg on cardiovascular outcomes [13]. With the current evidence, it is recommended to aim for home SBP <140 mmHg and inter-dialytic ASBP < 130 mmHg as these are associated with better outcomes in patients on hemodialysis [5, 14].

For measurement of outside-dialysis-unit BP, most studies monitored ambulatory BP and home BP for 44 hours and 7 days, respectively. However, it is acceptable to measure ABP for any 6-hour interval during the first 24 hours and home BP for 4 days after the midweek dialysis as these can provide similar prognostic values. Home BP measurements after the mid-week dialysis, including the weekend, had better prognostic significance than those on the first inter-dialytic day [15].

Treatment of Hypertension

Similar to the general population, hypertension in dialysis patients can be treated by antihypertensive medications as well as nonpharmacological measures.

Nonpharmacological Measures

Non-pharmacological measures are recommended to be the first step in lowering the BP in dialysis patients before initiation or titration of antihypertensive medications. These include dietary sodium restriction, enhanced sodium removal with dialysis, sodium matching and probing of dry weight [14]. Matching the dialysate sodium bath with pre-dialysis plasma sodium level can lower pre-dialysis BP by -15.6/-6.5 mmHg in patients with uncontrolled hypertension, but not in those with well-controlled hypertension at the baseline [16]. Volume overload can lead to uncontrolled hypertension in patients with ESRD and lowering of dry weight can effectively improve the intra-dialytic hypertension [17]. Duration and intensity of dialysis treatment are essential in achieving optimal dry weight. Shorter dialysis duration can hamper effective ultrafiltration [18] whereas more frequent or prolonged duration of dialysis treatment is more effective in achieving euvolemia and improving BP control [19].

Pharmacological Measures

Frequently, non-pharmacological measures alone are inadequate to control hypertension in dialysis patients. Antihypertensive medications are necessary to optimize BP control [6]. Unlike the general population, there are limited data in head to head comparison of antihypertensive medications to evaluate the cardiovascular advantage and mortality. The choice of antihypertensive medications depend on their side effects, tolerability of these side effects by the individuals, pharmacokinetics of the medications and underlying co-morbidities of the individuals [20]. Due to high pill burden and high rates of noncompliance among dialysis population, it is preferable to use formulations which require less frequent dosing. It is recommended to take daily dosing medications at nighttime to minimize the risk of intradialytic hypotension and counteract nocturnal increase in BP that is commonly seen with ESRD population [7].

Beta-Blockers

The pharmacokinetics of the beta-blockers vary greatly. Some are easily dialyzable while some are not. Carvedilol, propranolol, bisoprolol and labetolol are not easily removed by hemodialysis, whereas others, such as atenolol and metoprolol, have high dialyzability [21]. Among the beta-blockers, initiation of highly dialyzable ones was found to be associated with 40% higher risk of death in the following 180 days, comparing to those who received less dialyzable beta-blockers (relative risk, 1.4; 95% confidence interval, 1.1 - 1.8; $P < 0.01$) in a propensity-matched population-based retrospective cohort study with >6000 chronic hemodialysis patients older than 66 years of age [22]. The increased mortality was not related to the excess risk of myocardial infarction or heart failure. However, causal relationship between dialyzability of beta-blockers and mortality cannot be determined from this study [22].

Overall, beta-blockers have been shown to be associated with better cardiovascular outcomes [23]. It was found to improve survival (24), left ventricular function, risk of all-cause hospitalization (HR, 0.44; 95% CI, 0.25 to 0.77) including admissions for worsening of heart failure, fatal myocardial infarctions, fatal strokes and mortality (HR, 0.51; 95% CI, 0.32 to 0.82) in hemodialysis patients with dilated cardiomyopathy [25].

Renin-Angiotensin System Inhibitors

Among the Renin-Angiotensin System (RAS) Inhibitors, all angiotensin converting enzyme inhibitors (ACEI), except fosinopril and trandolapril, are removed by hemodialysis, whereas Angiotensin Receptor Blockers (ARBs) are not easily dialyzable [21].

The evidence for cardiovascular protective effect of RAS inhibitors in dialysis patient population has mixed results. Although ARB was associated with reduction in cardiovascular mortality (RR = 0.79; $P = 0.005$) in DOPPS study [23], neither fosinopril nor irbesartan has demonstrated cardiovascular protective benefits beyond antihypertensive effect in randomized trials with hemodialysis patients [26, 27]. Similar result with no significant reduction in cardiovascular morbidity and mortality (pooled RR, 0.66; 95% CI, 0.35 to 1.25, $p = 0.20$) was noted in the meta-analysis of randomized trials among dialysis patients taking ACEI or ARB. Larger, high-quality trials may be able to show the cardiovascular benefits of ACEI and ARB beyond their antihypertensive effects [28].

Beta-Blocker versus RAAS Blockade

Beta-blockers have been shown to have more favorable results than RAAS blockade agents in the ESRD population. A randomized controlled trial comparing the antihypertensive and cardiovascular protective effects of atenolol and lisinopril was terminated prematurely due to significantly excess risk of serious cardiovascular events, such as myocardial infarction, stroke, hospitalized heart failure, and cardiovascular death, in the lisinopril group. Due to early termination, the study lacked the power to evaluate improvement in left ventricular mass index in between the two groups [29]. Similarly, atenolol was found to have better efficacy in improving arterial stiffness, a marker for cardiovascular disease, compared to lisinopril, in a randomized trial with 179 hemodialysis patients [30].

Calcium Channel Blockers

Calcium channel blockers is one of most commonly used antihypertensive medications in dialysis patient population. Their lack of dialyzability [21] and once a day dosing make them the preferred agents in terms of compliance. Comparing to placebo, calcium channel blockers also have survival advantage as well as cardioprotective effects [31, 32].

Mineralocorticoid Receptor Antagonist

Addition of mineralocorticoid receptor antagonists (MRA), such as spironolactone or eplerenone, was shown to reduce cardiovascular events and improve mortality in patients with or without heart failure [33, 34]. In the Dialysis Outcomes Heart Failure Aldactone Study, cardiovascular death or cardiovascular-related hospitalization and all-cause mortality were reduced by 62% (HR, 0.38; 95% CI, 0.17 to 0.83) and 67% (HR, 0.335; 95% CI: 0.162 to 0.693; $p = 0.003$), respectively, in spironolactone arm during the 3-year follow up period [33]. The ongoing ALdosterone Antagonist Chronic HEModialysis Interventional Survival Trial (ALCHEMIST) aims to explore the effect of spironolactone on nonfatal myocardial infarction, acute coronary syndrome, hospitalization for heart failure, nonfatal stroke, or cardiovascular death in hemodialysis patients.

However, usage of MRA has been limited due to the concern of safety and tolerability as it can lead to hyperkalemia, especially in patients with advanced chronic kidney disease. It is unclear if the side effects are dose-related. Completion of the ongoing Safety and Cardiovascular Efficacy of Spironolactone in Dialysis-Dependent ESRD Trial (SPin-D) should address these concerns.

Others

Other classes of antihypertensive agents, such as centrally acting alpha-agonist (clonidine), direct vasodilators (minoxidil and hydralazine), and alpha-adrenergic blockers, are also effective in lowering the BP in dialysis patients. However, these medications are not used as first-line agents due to the concern of side-effects and frequent dosing [20]. Even though diuretics are not effective in controlling hypertension in anuric patients, they can be beneficial for dialysis patients with residual renal function in controlling interdialytic fluid gain as well as BP [20].

HYPOTENSION

Hypotension during or immediately following dialysis is a common phenomenon, affecting 5-30% of all outpatient dialysis treatments. Intradialytic hypotension (IDH) not only interferes with the effective delivery of dialysis treatment, but also affects the patient's overall well-being and quality of life by causing debilitating symptoms such as cramps. IDH also carries a host of potential complications, ranging from dysrhythmias, cardiac and cerebral ischemia, fistula or graft thrombosis, and fluid overload related to difficult ultrafiltration and need for fluid boluses [35].

Patients who experienced >35% of IDH episodes in their treatments faced a higher hospital admission rates and mortality as well [2]. Flythe et al. demonstrated an association between intradialytic nadir systolic BP <90 mmHg and increased all-cause mortality [36].

Definition and Prevalence

IDH is defined by KDOQI guidelines as a decrease in systolic blood pressure by ≥20 mm Hg or a decrease in MAP by 10 mm Hg associated with symptoms, including abdominal discomfort, nausea, vomiting, muscle cramps, dizziness, and fainting [7]. The incidence of IDH during each session of hemodialysis ranges from 20% to 30% [37]. In a recent study, IDH is quite frequent (17.2%) in the outpatient dialysis settings but also varies among patients (0-100%) and dialysis facilities (11.1-25.8%) [2]. IDH may occur early (less than one hour of treatment), late (after one hour), or post-dialysis. The early onset of IDH before significant ultrafiltration may be related to reduction in vascular tone as measured by aortic pulse wave velocity [38].

Risk Factors

Some of the common risk factors for IDH include younger age <30 years of age, older age >70 years of age, diabetes status, left ventricular hypertrophy (LVH) and diastolic dysfunction, history of myocardial infarction and coronary heart disease, large interdialytic weight gain (IDWG) >3% of body weight, anuria, autonomic dysfunction, hypoalbuminemia, longer dialysis vantage, and severe anemia [39, 2].

A Portugal study suggested that large IDWG may be a risk factor for IDH by demonstrating that the odds of IDH is 60% more likely on the first dialysis session of the week [40].

Causes of Intradialytic Hypotension

Most commonly, IDH occurs in the absence of serious acute conditions. However, it can be due to serious underlying medical conditions or a confluence of contributing factors rather than a single cause. Table 1 tabulates the common and uncommon causes of IDH.

Autonomic Dysfunction

Autonomic dysfunction occurs in over 50% of patients on maintenance dialysis and may contribute to intra-and-inter-dialytic hypotension [41]. It is usually due to the inability of baroreceptors to trigger release of catecholamine that promotes vasoconstriction in response to fluid removal [42].

Excessive Ultrafiltration (UF) Rate

A dialysis patient with volume overload often requires large UF to achieve the estimated dry weight during the typically prescribed 3-4 hours dialysis duration. As the rate of UF exceeds the rate of vascular filling, early hypovolemia sets in. This will activate the carotid baroreceptors and cause the ventricular wall mechanoreceptors to decrease firing, resulting in increased sympathetic activation to raise the blood pressure. But as more volume is removed, the ventricles contract more vigorously around a poorly filled LV cavity. This will paradoxically cause the ventricular wall mechanoreceptors to increase firing and inhibit the sympathetic baroreceptor reflex, leading to bradycardia, vasodilation, and hypotension.

Most patients can tolerate higher UF rate during early phase of dialysis since most of the excess fluid is in central circulation. As dialysis is continued, the rate of vascular filling may fall below the UF rate as most of the excess fluid is in the interstitial space. Large volume UF may thus overwhelm the compensatory mechanisms of vasoconstriction and increased cardiac output, resulting in IDH [37].

Table 1. Causes of Intradialytic Hypotension

Common Causes	Uncommon Causes
Intake of Antihypertensive Medications	Sepsis
Foods before dialysis	Arrhythmia
Excess Ultrafiltration	Cardiac Tamponade
Incorrect Target Dry Weight	Severe Heart Failure
Autonomic Dysfunction	Severe Valvular Disorders
Reduced Cardiac Function	Hemolysis
Rapid Reduction in Serum Osmolality due to high predialysis urea level	Pulmonary Embolism
	Air Embolism
	Dialyzer Reaction

Impaired Cardiac Function

Left ventricular hypertrophy (LVH) is common among dialysis patients and those with reduced cardiac reserves are at high risk for IDH [43, 44]. LVH leads to reduction on cardiac compliance that can cause significant decrease in cardiac output even with low UF rate. When compared to hypotension-resistant patients, hypotension-prone patients have less increase in cardiac index on dobutamine stress echocardiography. Repeated episodes of IDH may also induce ischemia-driven myocardial stunning that in turn further increase the risk of IDH [45].

Consequences of IDH

IDH carries a host of pathophysiological consequences, including reduced clearance of uremic toxins from interruption of effective dialysis delivery, ischemia-induced myocardial stunning, cerebrovascular ischemia, as well as cardiovascular morbidity [36, 46]. Recurrent IDH also accelerate loss of residual renal function through repeated episodes of renal ischemia [47].

Management of Intradialytic Hypotension

Nonpharmacologic Measures

Nonpharmacologic interventions (Table 2) are the mainstay of treatment for IDH. In addition to these conservative measures, patients with persistent IDH will need a cardiac evaluation, including an echocardiogram.

Salt Restriction

Patients prone to develop IDH should restrict their salt intake to avoid excessive IDWG. It has been estimated that an anuric dialysis patient will gain 1 liter of fluid for every 8 g of salt consumed. In a cross-sectional study, restricting salt intake to <5 g/day has been shown to lower IDWG, reduce frequency of IDH, as well as decrease left ventricular mass [48].

Table 2. Non-pharmacological Treatment for IDH

Acute Management
Immediate reduction or discontinuation of ultrafiltration
Administration of fluid bolus
Oxygen
Trendelenburg position to increase cerebral perfusion
Long Term Conservative Management
Reassessment of Estimated Dry Weight
Withholding antihypertensive medications before dialysis treatment
Avoiding food intake just before and during dialysis
Salt restriction
Reducing large IDWG
Cool-temperature dialysate

Cool-Temperature Dialysate

Cool-temperature hemodialysis is usually performed by reducing the dialysate temperature to 0.5 to 1.0 C below the patient's body temperature. Cold temperature dialysate promotes vasoconstriction and enhanced cardiac contractility through activation of the sympathetic nervous system. Its positive effect on blood pressure has been shown in a systematic review of 22 studies. The use of cool-temperature dialysate was associated with 7.1 times less frequent episodes of IDH [49]. Another meta-analysis in 2016 reconfirms the effectiveness of cool temperature dialysis on reducing IDH. In this meta study of 26 trials involving more than 484 patients, cool-temperature dialysate reduced the risk of intradialytic hypotension by 68 percent [50]. On the downside, patients on cool-temperature dialysis were 2.95 times more likely to experience the undesirable effects of feeling cold, shivering, or cramps.

Reducing UF Rate

A higher UF rate of > 13 ml/kg/hour is associated with increased all-cause and CVS-related mortality [17]. To minimize IDH and cardiovascular risk, some authors recommend fluid removal rates of ≤10 mL/kg/hour while acknowledging that this may be challenging in the in-center setting, especially in patients with large IDWG [51]. In those challenging cases, restricting IDWG (always conflict-fraught, often unachievable) or extending treatment duration to allow additional fluid removal time can be able to limit volume removal to ≤ 10 mL/kg/hour while still achieving euvolemia.

Pharmacologic Measures

Midodrine is a selective alpha-1 adrenergic agonist that has been successfully used to treat neurogenic causes of orthostatic hypotension. Prior small studies have also demonstrated the effectiveness of midodrine at improving BP stability during hemodialysis among patients with intradialytic hypotension [52]. While midodrine is a useful adjunctive therapy for IDH, it has significant side effects, including pruritus, gastrointestinal discomfort, supine hypertension, and urinary retention [53]. Patients with severe coronary artery disease should use midodrine with caution.

The authors have no financial conflicts of interest or grant support to declare.

This review has not been previously published.

References

[1] Agarwal R, Lewis RR. Prediction of hypertension in chronic hemodialysis patients. *Kidney Int*. 2001 Nov;60(5):1982–9.

[2] Sands JJ, Usvyat LA, Sullivan T, Segal JH, Zabetakis P, Kotanko P, et al. Intradialytic hypotension: frequency, sources of variation and correlation with clinical outcome. *Hemodial Int Int Symp Home Hemodial*. 2014 Apr;18(2):415–22.

[3] Agarwal R, Peixoto AJ, Santos SFF, Zoccali C. Pre- and postdialysis blood pressures are imprecise estimates of interdialytic ambulatory

blood pressure. *Clin J Am Soc Nephrol CJASN*. 2006 May;1(3): 389–98.

[4] Agarwal R. Blood pressure and mortality among hemodialysis patients. *Hypertens Dallas Tex* 1979. 2010 Mar;55(3):762–8.

[5] Alborzi P, Patel N, Agarwal R. Home blood pressures are of greater *prognostic value* than hemodialysis unit recordings. *Clin J Am Soc Nephrol* CJASN. 2007 Nov;2(6):1228–34.

[6] Agarwal R. Interdialytic hypertension-an update. *Adv Chronic Kidney Dis*. 2011 Jan;18(1):11–6.

[7] K/DOQI Workgroup. K/DOQI clinical practice guidelines for cardiovascular disease in dialysis patients. *Am J Kidney Dis Off J Natl Kidney Found.* 2005 Apr;45(4 Suppl 3):S1-153.

[8] Kalantar-Zadeh K, Kilpatrick RD, McAllister CJ, Greenland S, Kopple JD. Reverse epidemiology of hypertension and cardiovascular death in the hemodialysis population: the 58th annual fall conference and scientific sessions. *Hypertens Dallas Tex* 1979. 2005 Apr;45(4):811–7.

[9] Georgianos PI, Agarwal R. Blood pressure in hemodialysis: targets? *Curr Opin Nephrol Hypertens.* 2017 Aug 21;

[10] Georgianos PI, Agarwal R. Blood Pressure and Mortality in Long-Term Hemodialysis-Time to Move Forward. *Am J Hypertens*. 2017 Mar 1;30(3):211–22.

[11] Heerspink HJL, Ninomiya T, Zoungas S, de Zeeuw D, Grobbee DE, Jardine MJ, et al. Effect of lowering blood pressure on cardiovascular events and mortality in patients on dialysis: a systematic review and meta-analysis of randomised controlled trials. *Lancet Lond Engl.* 2009 Mar 21;373(9668):1009–15.

[12] Bansal N, McCulloch CE, Rahman M, Kusek JW, Anderson AH, Xie D, et al. Blood pressure and risk of all-cause mortality in advanced chronic kidney disease and hemodialysis: the chronic renal insufficiency cohort study. *Hypertens Dallas Tex* 1979. 2015 Jan;65(1):93–100.

[13] Gul A, Miskulin D, Gassman J, Harford A, Horowitz B, Chen J, et al. Design of the Blood Pressure Goals in Dialysis pilot study. *Am J Med Sci*. 2014 Feb;347(2):125–30.

[14] Agarwal RL. Debate from the 2012 ASH Annual Scientific Sessions: should blood pressure be reduced in hemodialysis patients? Pro position. *J Am Soc Hypertens JASH*. 2012 Dec;6(6):439–42.

[15] Agarwal R, Andersen MJ, Light RP. Location not quantity of blood pressure measurements predicts mortality in hemodialysis patients. *Am J Nephrol*. 2008;28(2):210–7.

[16] de Paula FM, Peixoto AJ, Pinto LV, Dorigo D, Patricio PJM, Santos SFF. Clinical consequences of an individualized dialysate sodium prescription in hemodialysis patients. *Kidney Int*. 2004 Sep;66(3):1232–8.

[17] Agarwal R, Light RP. Intradialytic hypertension is a marker of volume excess. *Nephrol Dial Transplant Off Publ Eur Dial Transpl Assoc - Eur Ren Assoc*. 2010 Oct;25(10):3355–61.

[18] Tandon T, Sinha AD, Agarwal R. Shorter delivered dialysis times associate with a higher and more difficult to treat blood pressure. *Nephrol Dial Transplant Off Publ Eur Dial Transpl Assoc - Eur Ren Assoc*. 2013 Jun;28(6):1562–8.

[19] Kotanko P, Garg AX, Depner T, Pierratos A, Chan CT, Levin NW, et al. Effects of frequent hemodialysis on blood pressure: Results from the randomized frequent hemodialysis network trials. *Hemodial Int Int Symp Home Hemodial*. 2015 Jul;19(3):386–401.

[20] *R GP and A. Pharmacotherapy of Hypertension in Chronic Dialysis Patients. - PubMed* - NCBI [Internet]. [cited 2017 Oct 27]. Available from: https://www.ncbi.nlm.nih.gov/pubmed/?term=Georgianos%2C+P.I.+and+R.+Agarwal%2C+Pharmacotherapy+of+Hypertension+in+Chronic+Dialysis+Patients.

[21] Inrig JK. Antihypertensive agents in hemodialysis patients: a current perspective. *Semin Dial*. 2010 Jun;23(3):290–7.

[22] Weir MA, Dixon SN, Fleet JL, Roberts MA, Hackam DG, Oliver MJ, et al. β-Blocker dialyzability and mortality in older patients receiving hemodialysis. *J Am Soc Nephrol JASN*. 2015 Apr;26(4):987–96.

[23] Lopes AA, Bragg-Gresham JL, Ramirez SPB, Andreucci VE, Akiba T, Saito A, et al. Prescription of antihypertensive agents to haemodialysis patients: time trends and associations with patient characteristics, country and survival in the DOPPS. *Nephrol Dial Transplant Off Publ Eur Dial Transpl Assoc - Eur Ren Assoc*. 2009 Sep;24(9):2809–16.

[24] Foley RN, Herzog CA, Collins AJ, United States Renal Data System. Blood pressure and long-term mortality in United States hemodialysis patients: USRDS Waves 3 and 4 Study. *Kidney Int.* 2002 Nov;62(5):1784–90.

[25] Cice G, Ferrara L, D'Andrea A, D'Isa S, Di Benedetto A, Cittadini A, et al. Carvedilol increases two-year survivalin dialysis patients with dilated cardiomyopathy: a prospective, placebo-controlled trial. *J Am Coll Cardiol.* 2003 May 7;41(9):1438–44.

[26] Zannad F, Kessler M, Lehert P, Grünfeld JP, Thuilliez C, Leizorovicz A, et al. Prevention of cardiovascular events in end-stage renal disease: results of a randomized trial of fosinopril and implications for future studies. *Kidney Int*. 2006 Oct;70(7):1318–24.

[27] Peters CD, Kjaergaard KD, Jensen JD, Christensen KL, Strandhave C, Tietze IN, et al. No significant effect of angiotensin II receptor blockade on intermediate cardiovascular end points in hemodialysis patients. *Kidney Int*. 2014 Sep;86(3):625–37.

[28] Tai DJ, Lim TW, James MT, Manns BJ, Tonelli M, Hemmelgarn BR, et al. Cardiovascular effects of angiotensin converting enzyme inhibition or angiotensin receptor blockade in hemodialysis: a meta-analysis. *Clin J Am Soc Nephrol CJASN*. 2010 Apr;5(4):623–30.

[29] Agarwal R, Sinha AD, Pappas MK, Abraham TN, Tegegne GG. Hypertension in hemodialysis patients treated with atenolol or lisinopril: a randomized controlled trial. *Nephrol Dial Transplant Off Publ Eur Dial Transpl Assoc - Eur Ren Assoc*. 2014 Mar;29(3): 672–81.

[30] Georgianos PI, Agarwal R. Effect of lisinopril and atenolol on aortic stiffness in patients on hemodialysis. *Clin J Am Soc Nephrol CJASN*. 2015 Apr 7;10(4):639–45.

[31] Tepel M, Hopfenmueller W, Scholze A, Maier A, Zidek W. Effect of amlodipine on cardiovascular events in hypertensive haemodialysis patients. *Nephrol Dial Transplant Off Publ Eur Dial Transpl Assoc - Eur Ren Assoc*. 2008 Nov;23(11):3605–12.

[32] Kestenbaum B, Gillen DL, Sherrard DJ, Seliger S, Ball A, Stehman-Breen C. Calcium channel blocker use and mortality among patients with end-stage renal disease. *Kidney Int*. 2002 Jun;61(6):2157–64.

[33] Matsumoto Y, Mori Y, Kageyama S, Arihara K, Sugiyama T, Ohmura H, et al. Spironolactone reduces cardiovascular and cerebrovascular morbidity and mortality in hemodialysis patients. *J Am Coll Cardiol*. 2014 Feb 18;63(6):528–36.

[34] Lin C, Zhang Q, Zhang H, Lin A. Long-Term Effects of Low-Dose Spironolactone on Chronic Dialysis Patients: A Randomized Placebo-Controlled Study. *J Clin Hypertens Greenwich Conn*. 2016 Feb;18(2):121–8.

[35] Stefánsson BV, Brunelli SM, Cabrera C, Rosenbaum D, Anum E, Ramakrishnan K, et al. Intradialytic hypotension and risk of cardiovascular disease. *Clin J Am Soc Nephrol CJASN*. 2014 Dec 5;9(12):2124–32.

[36] Flythe JE, Xue H, Lynch KE, Curhan GC, Brunelli SM. Association of mortality risk with various definitions of intradialytic hypotension. *J Am Soc Nephrol JASN*. 2015 Mar;26(3):724–34.

[37] Daugirdas JT. Pathophysiology of dialysis hypotension: an update. *Am J Kidney Dis Off J Natl Kidney Found*. 2001 Oct;38(4 Suppl 4):S11-17.

[38] Power A, Charitaki E, Davenport A. Changes in Vascular Tone Occur Early During Hemodialysis Treatments Independently of Volume Reduction. *Artif Organs*. 2016 Jul;40(7):678–83.

[39] Schreiber MJ. Setting the stage. *Am J Kidney Dis Off J Natl Kidney Found*. 2001 Oct;38(4 Suppl 4):S1–10.

[40] Rocha A, Sousa C, Teles P, Coelho A, Xavier E. Effect of Dialysis Day on Intradialytic Hypotension Risk. *Kidney Blood Press Res*. 2016;41(2):168–74.

[41] Ewing DJ, Winney R. Autonomic function in patients with chronic renal failure on intermittent haemodialysis. *Nephron.* 1975;15(6): 424–9.

[42] Daul AE, Wang XL, Michel MC, Brodde OE. Arterial hypotension in chronic hemodialyzed patients. *Kidney Int.* 1987 Nov;32(5):728–35.

[43] Poldermans D, Man in 't Veld AJ, Rambaldi R, Van Den Meiracker AH, Van Den Dorpel MA, Rocchi G, et al. Cardiac evaluation in hypotension-prone and hypotension-resistant hemodialysis patients. *Kidney Int.* 1999 Nov;56(5):1905–11.

[44] Foley RN, Parfrey PS, Harnett JD, Kent GM, Martin CJ, Murray DC, et al. Clinical and echocardiographic disease in patients starting end-stage renal disease therapy. *Kidney Int.* 1995 Jan;47(1):186–92.

[45] Burton JO, Jefferies HJ, Selby NM, McIntyre CW. Hemodialysis-induced cardiac injury: determinants and associated outcomes. *Clin J Am Soc Nephrol CJASN.* 2009 May;4(5):914–20.

[46] McIntyre CW, Goldsmith DJ. Ischemic brain injury in hemodialysis patients: which is more dangerous, hypertension or intradialytic hypotension? *Kidney Int.* 2015 Jun;87(6):1109–15.

[47] Wong J, Vilar E, Davenport A, Farrington K. Incremental haemodialysis. *Nephrol Dial Transplant Off Publ Eur Dial Transpl Assoc - Eur Ren Assoc.* 2015 Oct;30(10):1639–48.

[48] Kayikcioglu M, Tumuklu M, Ozkahya M, Ozdogan O, Asci G, Duman S, et al. The benefit of salt restriction in the treatment of end-stage renal disease by haemodialysis. *Nephrol Dial Transplant Off Publ Eur Dial Transpl Assoc - Eur Ren Assoc.* 2009 Mar;24(3):956–62.

[49] Selby NM, McIntyre CW. A systematic review of the clinical effects of reducing dialysate fluid temperature. *Nephrol Dial Transplant Off Publ Eur Dial Transpl Assoc - Eur Ren Assoc.* 2006 Jul;21(7): 1883–98.

[50] *Effect of Lowering the Dialysate Temperature in Chronic Hemodialysis: A Systematic Review and Meta-Analysis. - PubMed - NCBI* [Internet]. [cited 2017 Dec 6]. Available from: https:// www.ncbi.nlm.nih.gov/pubmed/?term=Effect+of+Lowering+the+Dia

lysate+Temperature+in+Chronic+Hemodialysis%3A+A+Systematic +Review+and+Meta-Analysis.

[51] Agar JWM. Personal viewpoint: Limiting maximum ultrafiltration rate as a potential new measure of dialysis adequacy. *Hemodial Int Int Symp Home Hemodial.* 2016 Jan;20(1):15–21.

[52] Lin YF., Wang JY, Denq JC., Lin SH. Midodrine improves chronic hypotension in hemodialysis patients. *Am J Med Sci.* 2003 May;325(5):256–61.

[53] Izcovich A, González Malla C, Manzotti M, Catalano HN, Guyatt G. Midodrine for orthostatic hypotension and recurrent reflex syncope: A systematic review. *Neurology*. 2014 Sep 23;83(13):1170–7.

In: Advances in Health and Disease. Volume 4 ISBN: 978-1-53613-345-5
Editor: Lowell T. Duncan

Chapter 9

IMPROVING HEALTH AND WELL-BEING THROUGH CLIMATE CHANGE ADAPTATION

Peni H. Havea**, *Sarah L. Hemstock, PhD and Helene Jacot Des Combes, PhD
PaCE-SD, The University of the South Pacific, Suva, Fiji

ABSTRACT

Understanding the perceptions of climate change impacts on people's health and well-being in coastal communities is essential to develop adaptation strategies that will improve the health and well-being of community members in coastal areas. Here, an integrated mixed method approach: concurrent convergence parallel triangulation design – was used in 5 coastal communities in Tongatapu, Tonga. Community members were interviewed. Some of them had their health and well-being affected by climate change and some were not affected. Their responses were analyzed using a non-parametric test – chi-square analysis. Themes regarding the impact of climate change on health and well-being were then used to generate a further hypothesis. The results show that those whose health and well-being was affected differed significantly from those who were

* Corresponding Author Email: ilaisiaimoana@yahoo.com.

unaffected. They also indicated that all aspects of well-being: physical, mental and spiritual were affected by climate change and that people were eager to see the implementation of climate change adaptation strategies to improve their health and restore their mental well-being. It is thus essential to include these issues in adaptation strategies to ensure that local people are supporting and taking ownership of their resilience building.

Keywords: Tonga, health, well-being, climate change adaptation

1. INTRODUCTION

According to the World Risk Index report United Nation University (Institute for Environment and Human Security) (2016) report, Tonga was identified as the second most at risk country in the world, especially because of its coastal areas and communities that are affected negatively by disasters caused by natural hazards. This risk will exacerbate as the 5th Assessment Reports produced by the Inter-Governmental Panel on Climate Change (IPCC) (IPCC, 2014a; 2014b) have projected, that the negative impacts of climate change are likely to increase. Since damages to people's livelihoods, health and well-being caused by climate change impacts and disasters caused by natural hazards (Food and Agriculture Organisation (FAO) & Ministry of Agriculture Food Forests and Fisheries (MAFFF), 2014; Government of Tonga & UNDP, 2009; Ministry of Environment and Climate Change & National Emergency Management Office, 2010; Reddy, 1983; The Pacific Islands Regional Climate Assessment (PIRCA), 2012; United Nation University (Institute for Environment and Human Security), 2016; WHO, 2015; Woodroffe, 1983) are expected to be permanent for Tonga (ADB, 2016; Government of Tonga, 2015; Ministry of Environment and Climate Change & National Emergency Management Office, 2010), this paper assesses the perceptions of climate change impacts in five coastal communities in Tongatapu, Tonga: Kanokupolu, 'Ahau, Tukutonga, Popua and Manuka. The results from this study are expected to help the implementation of the nation's roadmap to building a resilient Tonga, by

2035 and beyond (Government of Tonga, 2016), thus helping the people in their own communities, managing the impacts of climate change better.

To achieve this goal, the perceptions of 460 participants have been evaluated, based on a convergence model that includes element derived from both quantitative and qualitative studies. This design allowed to differentiate those who were affected and those who were not. It was expected that those whose health and well-being was affected would differ significantly from those who were not (Casimiro, Calheiros, Santos, & Kovats, 2006; Creswell, 2013; 2014; Creswell & Plano Clark, 2007; 2011; Ebi, Kovats, & Menne, 2006; Grasso, Manera, Chiabai, & Markandya, 2012; Kovats, Menne, Ahern, & Patz, 2003; Senbeta, 2009; Wasswa, 2010).

This impact assessment would help people to improve their health and well-being through climate change adaptation, thus helping Tonga to achieve its target to address UNFCCC, UNCBD, UNCCD, IPCC and SDGs in its national development strategy, thus contributing significantly in making Tonga a more resilient and sustainable nation.

2. Methods

2.1. Study Sample

The overarching goal of the study was to provide a better understanding of the impact of climate change on health and well-being of Tongans aged 15 to 75 in Kanokupolu, ‘Ahau, Tukutonga, Popua and Manuka. The design of the study was a *Concurrent Convergence Parallel Triangulation Design* of 460 Tongans aged 15 to 75 in 5 coastal communities in Tongatapu. We called it *concurrent* because we collected the data at the same time frame. Then, there was a *convergence* in the sense that quantitative and qualitative studies were merged in the design phase as well as the analytical phase. The study was *parallel* because qualitative and quantitative data were weighted equally – with no emphasis at all. And there was *triangulation* since more than one method was used to collect the data. The studied participants were selected for IDI (in-depth interview) and FGD (focus group discussion) using a simple randomization technique (Creswell & Plano Clark, 2007; 2011). From the 460 participants who had completed a structured questionnaire, 28 were then randomly selected to do FGD and 24 for IDI. KII (key informant interview) of 12 participants older than 75 years old, government officials and church ministers were then carried out to supplement the study. The study protocols were approved by PaCE-SD and funded by the Research Office at USP under its Regional Ph.D. Scholarship Funding scheme.

2.2. Reliability Statistics for Health and Well-Being Impacts

In addition to information obtained from respondents on age and Christianity, information was also collected on the impact of climate change on health and well-being, via a self-administered questionnaire with a 5-point Likert scale: strongly disagree, disagree, neutral, agree, strongly agree and nominal measures: yes and no.

Reliability analysis of the questions for the Likert questionnaire was carried out to verify the validity and consistency of the scale used to measure climate change impacts on health and well-being item in this study. Reliability statistics were calculated, using 4 variables (Q83, Q84, Q93, Q94) out of 109 questions sorted by measurement for health and well-being affected. Climate change impact on health and well-being of Tongans aged 15 to 75 on 5 coastal communities in Tongatapu appeared to have an adequate internal consistency, $\alpha = .745$. An adequate threshold for internal consistency is .7 (Pochampally & Gupta, 2016).

2.3. IDI, KII and FGD

The researcher carried out IDI, KII and trained professional facilitators organized the FGD. These interviews and focus groups were recorded, transcribed, and entered into Nvivo10 software for coding and analysis

(Miles & Huberman, 1994; Miles, Huberman, & Saldaña, 2014; QSR International, 2014). The interview and focus group questions were used to examine participants perceptions of the impact of climate change on their health and well-being. Because perceived impacts of climate change on a person's health and well-being are complex, the questionnaire did not include simple questions yes-or-no response. The interviewer probed further to ensure the participant's discussion focuses on impacts of climate change or also included different stressors. In summary, a myriad of impact conditions on health and well-being, for example, asthma, stress and anxiety, have been captured using convergent model.

2.4. Data Analysis

The data analytic strategy reflects the integration of hypothesis testing and hypothesis generation in a single study that is the hallmark of using concurrent convergence parallel triangulation design. In the first phase, participants who were affected by climate change and those who were not were compared using χ^2 or chi-square goodness-of-fit, respectively.

The level of statistical significance was set at $\alpha = .05$, recognizing that tests of statistical significance are approximations that serves as a catalyst that facilitates interpretation and inference. In the second phase, a constant comparative analysis was used, moving iteratively between codes and texts to derive themes related to the impact of climate change on health and well-being (Creswell, 2013; 2014; Miles & Huberman, 1994; Miles et al., 2014).

Then, the convergence design was used to take 1 theme from the data and comparing it with the survey data that may be of similar, to develop a conceptualization and/or a better understanding of those whose perceived health and well-being were affected from those who were not (Table 1). Data analysis was carried out with the use of SPSS 24 (IBM Corporation, New York, USA), Nvivo 10 (QSR International, Victoria, Australia), r studio 1.0.153 and python 3.6.

3. RESULTS

3.1. Study Population Pyramid

The study has surveyed more females (53%) than males (47%) with a ratio of 61:54, female to male participants (Figure 1). The most important point to note is that although the sample included a large number of young people, it has also spread across the age range to include also 65-75 years old. This pyramid is almost comparable with the total population of Tonga in the 2016 census (Statistic Department of Tonga, 2016). The mean age was 25-34 years old (35.9%) with a χ^2 (5) = 155.91, p < .000. The number of Christianity was 460 (100%).

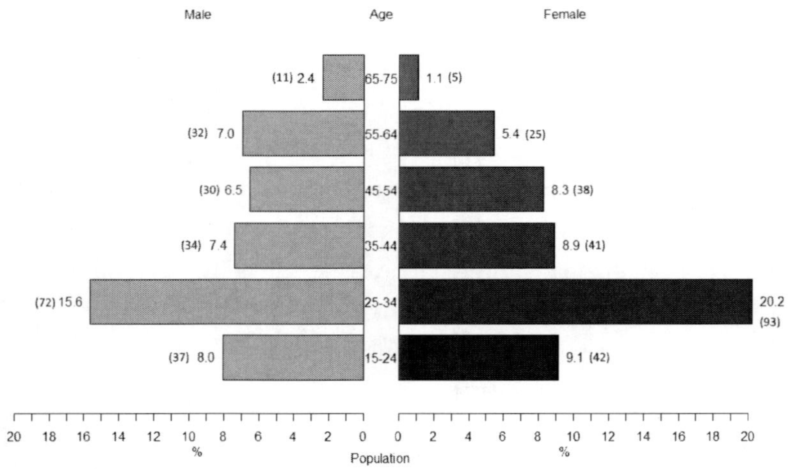

Figure 1. Study population pyramid, 2013.

3.2. Population Pyramid Plot for Health and Well-Being affected

Based on this sample, 9 in 10 of the respondents have indicated that their health and well-being were affected by climate change impacts (Figure 2). Because of this high figure, improving health and well-being through climate change adaptation is therefore needed for these 5 coastal communities and Tonga as a country.

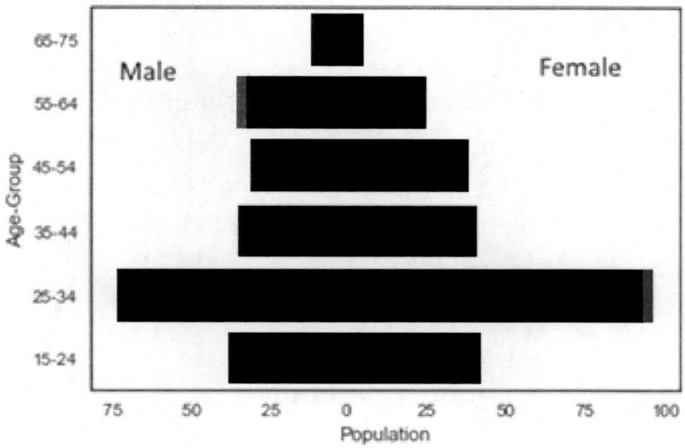

(a) People who have indicated that their health was affected by climate change. The dark grey color indicates 'health not affected' and the black color corresponds to 'health affected'.

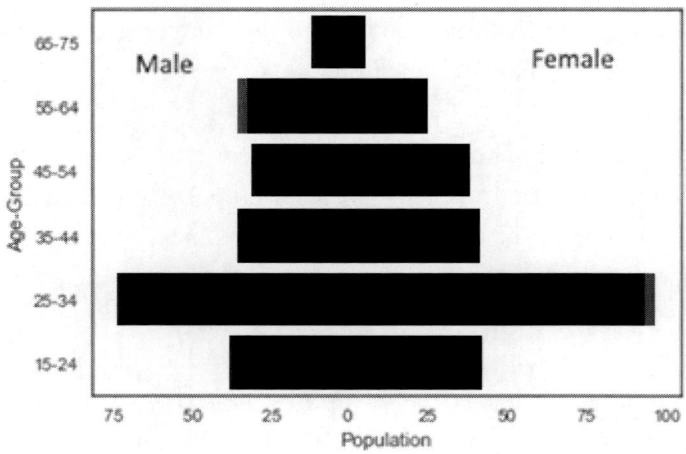

(b) People who have indicated that their well-being was affected by climate change. The dark grey color indicates 'well-being not affected' and the black color corresponds to 'well-being affected'.

Figure 2. Number of people whose health and well-being was affected by climate change.

3.3. Chi-square Goodness of Fit for Health and Well-Being Affected

Comparison of participants whose perceived health and well-being were affected differed significantly from those who were unaffected (Table 1). Those whose health and well-being was not affected did not experience health problems like asthma amongst others and well-being impacts such as physical, mental and spiritual impacts.

3.4. Themes Emerged in Interviews and FGD

Two themes that emerged from a careful review of the transcripts were selected for their climate change impacts and adaptation importance. The themes were related to the perceptions of impacts of climate change on health and well-being amongst Tongans aged 15 to 75 in Kanokupolu, ‘Ahau, Tukutonga, Popua and Manuka and their importance to improving them through climate change adaptation.

3.4.1. ‘Health Impact’ Vs Health Not Affected

This theme emerged from participants who perceived climate change has impacts on human or on a person’s health. These perceived impacts include shortness of breath (59.1%), asthma (41.3%), influenza (38.9%), pneumonia (20%), and other diseases (Table 1). For instance, a female participant from Kanokupolu said: “The only time that I usually get sick is when there is climate change like a little bit hotter. Sometimes warming climate usually got me sick so easily like flu viral illness, asthma, and shortness of breath. And it usually happened somewhere around November, December up to February during our wet seasons. During these times of the year, I usually get those illnesses. And even nowadays, I felt that climate change is getting worse, because it feels even hotter, during days and at night times. And especially flu, common cold, coughing and rhinorrhea, it usually affects me.”

Table 1. Impact on perceived health and well-being

Climate change impact indicator	Affected (Count, %)	Not affected (Count, %)	*P* Value
Health and well-being	382 (83.1%)	37 (8.1%)	.000
Health			
Overall	400 (87%)	60 (13%)	.000
Shortness of	272 (59.1%)	188 (40.9%)	.000
breath	190 (41.3%)	270 (58.7%)	.000
Asthma	179 (38.9%)	281 (61.1%)	.000
Influenza	92 (20%)	368 (80%)	.000
Pneumonia	<50 (10.8%)	>410 (89.1%)	.000
Others			
Well-being	397 (86.3%)	16 (3.5%)	.000
Overall	425 (92.4%)	6 (1.3%)	.000
Emotional	447 (97.2%)	13 (2.8%)	.000
Physical	448 (97.4%)	12 (2.6%)	.000
Mental	451 (98%)	9 (2%)	.000
Spiritual			

Those whose health was not affected stated that their health was fined. For example, a participant from Kanokupolu was saying that "I am a very healthy person."

3.4.2. 'Well-being Impact' Vs Well-Being Not Affected

This theme perceives how climate change affects mental well-being (97.4%), physical well-being (97.2%) and spiritual well-being (98%) of a person's overall well-being (86.3%) in the study (Table 1). For example, a male participant from Kanokupolu was saying: "Heavy rainfall for a very long period of time is not good for me, though, my families, and our overall well-being. The reason for this feeling of disappointment and stress is because I can't go to the bush to do my chores. When rainfall extended for almost a month, then, I have no choice, but to wear a raincoat or take an umbrella with me, and went straight to do my chores in our bushland. I just go up there to get us some food for our family and then come back home right away."

This excerpt shows the impacts of climate change on mental well-being and the same man concord it to impact on physical and spiritual well-being, who stated: "Schools kids and church were also affected when we had long-standing rainfall." A female participant from Manuka elaborates what the male participant from Kanokupolu stated above about impact on education and church and said: "I've always prioritized church to come first. I'm a preacher, and since, I was young I've always put God first. I am the principal of the Sunday school in our church, and we are the maintenance steward. Every day, I read my Bible, and always do my prayer in secret as in daily bread devotions. I have attended all the church services, although there will be climate change like rainfall and so on. Sometimes, however, I missed it due to some extreme natural events, but when I stayed home I can't sleep, rather I keep on reading the scriptures. I don't feel completely spiritually, fully occupied on that day, because I wanted to go to church and praise God by singing."

Those whose well-being was not affected stated that they are happy. For example, a female participant from Kanokupolu was saying: "Although I know that climate change is driven by nature and human-induced activities, I feel happy about it because our family overall well-being is satisfied. We get what we want in order to survive and make us happy."

4. Discussion

Our mixed approach combined survey questionnaire, interviews and FGD in a single study. Statistical tests did differentiate between participants whose health and well-being was affected and those who were not. When participants were asked to reflect on how climate change affects their health and well-being, two themes emerged. These themes represent participants' perceptions of the impacts of climate change on livelihoods, health and well-being.

'Health impact' depicts the notions that climate change has affected a person's health, negatively. The quantitative analysis showed that significant differences were found between participants who have had shortness of breath – 59.1% (272), asthma – 41.3% (190), influenza – 38.9% (179), pneumonia – 20% (92), and other diseases – <10.8% (50), like general malaise, CVD (cerebral vascular disease), sore throat, abdominal pain, filariasis, conjunctivitis, typhoid fever, skeletal pain, leptospirosis, dengue fever, diabetes, hypertension, back pain, CVA (cerebral vascular accident), gout arthritis, cancer, depression and anxiety, boils, gastroenteritis, fever, chest pain, poliomyelitis, epilepsy, anaphylaxis, cramps, STIs (sexually transmitted infections), urticaria, menorrhagia, migraine, pruritus, tinea, folliculitis, emesis, and those who were not. The same impacts on health that the WHO (2015) found such as diarrheal diseases and dengue fever for Tonga as well as other Pacific islanders – Cook Islands, Fiji, Kiribati, Marshall Islands, Micronesia, Nauru, Niue, Palau, Samoa, Solomon Islands, Tuvalu and Vanuatu.

A male participant from Manuka commented on how his health was affected by saying: "When climate change is happening, it affects me as a person" suggested that "When the weather is hot or cold, it causes me to have some kind of shortness of breath. I don't have any medical history like a known asthmatic disease, no, not at all. What I'm trying to say is that when the climate is changing it affects my aspiration in breathing". A woman from Manuka expresses her perception on the perceives linked between climate change and health: "When we had changing climate, my kids would have coughing and rhinorrhea, especially in cold season. This suggested, "I have these two little grandchildren of my eldest daughter, who have usually experienced shortness of breath in changing climate". Both health problems were concorded with the above quantitative assessment for asthma and shortness of breath.

'Well-being impact' then expressed by participants who perceived their well-being were affected by climate change, negatively. Our analytical approach shows that participants whom overall well-being (86.3%), emotional well-being (92.4%), physical well-being (97.2%), mental well-being (97.4%) and spiritual well-being (98%) were affected have differed significantly from those who were not. For example, people whose well-being were affected were getting sick (e.g., asthma and shortness of breath), stress and had anxiety when climate change was affecting them as well as not happy when they cannot be able to attend church due to some changing climate activities. As a male participant from Kanokupolu have stated: "…church was also affected when we had long-standing rainfall," suggested that spiritual well-being was affected by climate change. More importantly, our sample of 460 were all Christian (N = 460, 100%) by faith, regardless of the churches they go to, shows that not only Tonga is a Christian State, but how strong people relied on their God for protection. Those whose well-being were not affected are either healthy or happy with their lives.

Perceived health and well-being impacts are particularly acute in these five coastal communities in Tongatapu, Tonga and it is expected that these impacts will be exacerbated in the future, if communities do not build resilience in health and/or health and well-being adaptation programme that would allow them to cope with climate change better (National Academies of Sciences Engineering and Medicine, 2017).

Therefore, based on this analysis, a community-based health adaptation measure will be needed to improve the health and well-being of the people in these coastal communities. For example, the building of multi-purpose hall for these communities that could also be used as an evacuation center and health clinic will make people happy as they know that these safety measures are put in place to safeguard and protect their lives. Another example, is to ensure safety and clean water supply and community sanitation after cyclones or tsunamis, by storing enough water in a clean and a large container at home and clean their homes as soon as climate change and disasters finished.

Regarding well-being, a spiritual adaptation in the form of praying and/or fasting to their Christian God is expected to help to reverse these impacts from their communities in Tonga. Most importantly, as highlighted by the participant from Manuka, since Church is a powerful organization in the Tongan society, it may become an important stakeholder to perfect the course of adaptation better, thus complementing actions from the government and relevant stakeholders by tackling climate change at the community level.

As improving health and well-being through climate change adaptation is significant for the lives of the people in these communities, it should, therefore, be addressed in the Resilient Tonga policy for 2035 and beyond. Doing it this way will not only be making Tonga more resilient in their approach to adapt to the effects of climate change now and in the future, but it will also support Tonga to become a sustainable nation – as it will meet its localized Sustainable Development Goals (SDGs) (Government of Tonga, 2015) as well.

CONCLUSION

In conclusion, our findings have both community and methodological implications. For these coastal communities, it helps them strengthening and building safety and resilience measures to respond effectively. From a methodological perspective, if we limited the analysis to the participant's impact survey questionnaire per se, we would have missed the voices of the participants. As a result of this multimethodological approach, it is therefore recommended that people's health and well-being can be improved through climate change adaptation.

ACKNOWLEDGMENTS

We would like to thank the people of Kanokupolu, 'Ahau, Tukutonga, Popua and Manuka as well those from the Government of Tonga and Churches who were participated in the study. We want to also acknowledge PaCE-SD (Pacific Centre for Environment and Sustainable Development) for supervising this project and the Research Office at USP (The University of the South Pacific), for funding this work under its Ph.D. Regional Scholarship Fund, No. 6F004-3107-70766-00.

REFERENCES

ADB. (2016). *Validation Report - Tonga: Integrated urban development sector project* (No. 0108): Asian Development Bank - Independent Evaluation Department.

Casimiro, E., Calheiros, J., Santos, F. D., & Kovats, R. (2006). National assessment of human health effects of climate change in Portugal: approach and key findings. *Environ. Health Perspect., 114*(12), 1950-1956.

Creswell, J. W. (2013). *Qualitative inquiry and research design: Choosing among five approaches*. United State of America: SAGE.

Creswell, J. W. (2014). *Research Design*. Los Angeles: SAGE.

Creswell, J. W., & Plano Clark, V. L. (2007). *Designing and Conducting Mixed Methods Research*. United State of America: SAGE.

Creswell, J. W., & Plano Clark, V. L. (2011). *Designing and Conducting Mixed Methods Research* (2nd ed.). United State of America: SAGE.

Ebi, K. L., Kovats, R., & Menne, B. (2006). An approach for assessing human health vulnerability and public health interventions to adapt to climate change. *Environ. Health Perspect., 114*(12), 1930-1934. 10.1289/ehp.8430.

Food and Agriculture Organisation (FAO), & Ministry of Agriculture Food Forests and Fisheries (MAFFF). (2014). *Cyclone Ian in Ha'apai: Rapid damage assessment to the agriculture and fisheries sectors report*. Tonga: Ministry of Agriculture and Food, Forests and Fisheries.

Government of Tonga. (2015). *Tonga strategic development framework 2015-2025 - A more progressive Tonga: Enhancing our inheritance*. Tonga: Ministry of Finance and National Planning.

Government of Tonga. (2016). *Tonga climate change policy: A resilience Tonga by 2035*. Tonga: Government of Tonga.

Government of Tonga, & UNDP. (2009). *Tsunami recovery priority plan: Niuatoputapu Tonga*. Nuku'alofa: Government of Tonga.

Grasso, M., Manera, M., Chiabai, A., & Markandya, A. (2012). The health effects of climate change: A survey of recent quantitative research. *Int. J. Environ. Res. Public Health, 9*(5), 1523-1547.

IPCC. (2014a). *Climate Change 2014: Impacts, Adaptation, and Vulnerability. Part A: Global and Sectoral Aspects. Contribution of Working Group II to the Fifth Assessment Report of the Intergovernmental Panel on Climate Change*. Cambridge: Cambridge University Press.

IPCC. (2014b). *Climate Change 2014: Impacts, Adaptation, and Vulnerability. Part B: Regional Aspects. Contribution of Working Group II to the Fifth Assessment Report of the Intergovernmental Panel on Climate Change*. Cambridge: Cambridge University Press.

Kovats, R., Menne, B., Ahern, M., & Patz, J. (2003). National assessments of health impacts of climate change: *A review Climate change and human health: Risks and responses* (McMicheal AJ, Cambell-Lendrum D, Corvalan CF, Ebi KL, Gotheko A, Scheraga JD, Woodward A, eds). Geneva: WHO, World Meterological Organisation, United Nations Environment Programme.

Miles, M. B., & Huberman, A. M. (1994). *Qualitative Analysis: An Expanded Sourcebook* (2nd ed.). London SAGE.

Miles, M. B., Huberman, A. M., & Saldaña, J. (2014). *Qualitative Data Analysis: A Methods Sourcebook* (3rd ed.). London: SAGE.

Ministry of Environment and Climate Change, & National Emergency Management Office. (2010). *Tonga: Joint national action plan on climate change adaptation and disaster risk management 2010-2015.* Nuku'alofa: Kingdom of Tonga.

National Academies of Sciences Engineering and Medicine. (2017). *Protecting the Health and Well-Being of Communities in a Changing Climate: Proceedings of a Workshop*. The National Academies Press. https://doi.org/10.17226/24846.

Pochampally, K. K., & Gupta, S. M. (2016). *Reliability analysis with Minitab*. USA: CRC Press - Taylor & Francis Group.

QSR International. (2014). *Nvivo 10 for windows getting started.* Australia: QSR International Pty Ltd.

Reddy, S. D. (1983). *Tropical cyclone Isaac, 28 February 3 March 1982*. Fiji: Fiji Meteorological Service.

Senbeta, A. F. (2009). *Climate change impact on livelihoods, vulnerability and coping mechanisms: A case study on West-Arsi Zone, Ethiopia.* Unpublished Master, Lund University, Sweden.

Statistic Department of Tonga. (2016). *Tonga 2011 census of population and housing: Volume 1 - basic tables and administrative report*. Tonga: Tonga Department of Statistics.

The Pacific Islands Regional Climate Assessment (PIRCA). (2012). *Climate change and Pacific Islands: Indicators and impacts*. Washington: Island Press.

United Nation University (Institute for Environment and Human Security). (2016). *World risk report 2016: Focus (logistic and infrastructure)*. Tokyo, Japan: UNU.

Wasswa, F. N. (2010). *Climate change and livelihoods: Implications and evidences from Uganda.* Unpublished PhD, University of Pretoria, Pretoria (SA).

WHO. (2015). *Human health and climate change in Pacific Island countries*. Geneva: World Health Organisation.

Woodroffe, C. D. (1983). The Impact of Cyclone Isaac on the Coast of Tonga. *University of Hawaii Press, 37*(3), 181-210.

Biographical Sketch

Peni Hausia Havea

Affiliation: PaCE-SD, The University of the South Pacific, Suva, Fiji

Education: MPH, PhD in Climate Change [Finishing Candidate]

Research and Professional Experience: Climate change, livelihoods, health and well-being

In: Advances in Health and Disease. Volume 4 ISBN: 978-1-53613-345-5
Editor: Lowell T. Duncan

Chapter 10

ORAL HYGIENE AUTONOMY PROMOTION IN INDIVIDUALS WITH SPECIAL NEEDS

Maria Cristina Duarte Ferreira[1,*], DDS, PhD,
Bruna Sumaya Souza Pinto[2],
Manuela Costa Andrade Silva[2],
Sucena Matuk Long[1], DDS, PhD,
Renata Pilli Joias DDS[1], PhD
and Erika Josgrilberg Guimarães[1], DDS, PhD
[1]Pediatric Dentistry and Public Health Departments of Health and Medicine Science School of Universidade Metodista de São Paulo, Brazil
[2]Dentistry School of Universidade Metodista de São Paulo, Brazil

* Corresponding Author: Maria Cristina Duarte Ferreira, Professor; R. Cancioneiro de Évora, 24; CEP: 04708-010 – São Paulo – SP – Brazil; duarteferreira@uol.com.br.

ABSTRACT

This study aimed to verify the influence of different motivational interventions for oral hygiene autonomy promotion on the biofilm control in individuals with special needs. The study sample consisted of 21 adult individuals with mean age of 30 years, with several types of disabilities (cerebral palsy, Down syndrome, intellectual retarded, and autism), employees of the sector of artisan products of the Universidade Metodista de São Paulo. The biofilm was evaluated through the Simplified Oral Hygiene Index (OHI-S) proposed by Greene and Vermillion (1964). None of the participants (0%) exhibited excellent or bad initial values of oral hygiene; 80.95% exhibited good and 19.05% regular initial values. Then, four different types of motivational activities on oral health were carried out for 4 months. The following percentages of the values of oral hygiene after the first motivational activity (motivational theater) were observed: excellent and bad 0%, good 66.7%, and regular 33.33%. After the second motivational activity (group dynamics with sequence of tooth brushing play, none of the participants presented excellent OHI-S, while 23.8% scored regular, 71.4% good and 4.8% bad. In the motivational activity of supervised tooth brushing, we verified an increasing of good OHI-S (90.4%) and a decreasing for regular OHI-S (9.6%). The last motivational intervention was a talk with parents and/or guardians and the OHI-S analysis showed that 4.8% reached an excellent score, 90.4% a good score, 4.8% a regular score and 0% a bad score. The Friedman test ($p<0.005$) revealed statistically significant differences in the comparison between the 1st and 5th; 2nd and 4th; 2nd and 5th; 3rd and 4th; and 3rd and 5th OHI-S assessments. It was concluded that the oral hygiene promotion autonomy in individuals with special needs can be effective, especially when a continuous and individualized following-up is possible in addition to the motivation of parents and/or guardians. Thus, OHI-S decreased, ensuring an improvement in oral health. These data suggest that motivational activities can be developed to promote autonomy in other aspects of general health, resulting in the improvement of the quality of life of individuals with special needs.

Keywords: education, dental, dental plaque, quality of life

INTRODUCTION

Individuals with special needs exist worldwide. In Brazil, the last demographic census in 2010 showed that 23.9% of the total population presents some kind of impairment [1].

This figure has been increasing due to demographic growth, advancements in medicine and to the aging process. In countries where life expectancy is above 70 years of age, each individual will live, on average, for 8 years with a disability, or 11.5% of his or her existence. This data shows the importance of getting to know "the largest minority in the world" even better [2].

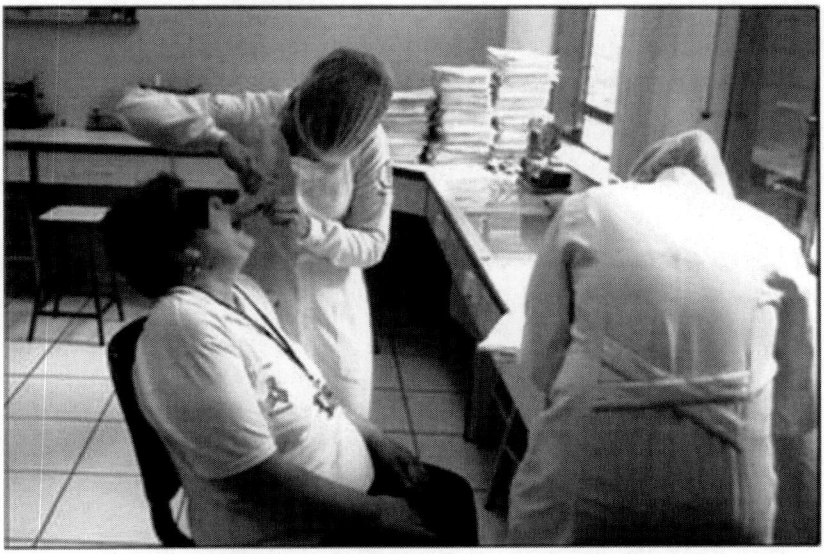

Figure 1. Oral clinical examination.

These individuals tend to present higher risks of developing tooth decay and gum disease. The physical and/or limitation level; the difficulty in carrying out oral hygiene; the diet, which is generally rich in carbohydrates and soft food because many times their oral hygiene is disregarded by their caregivers, are factors that stimulate the accumulation of bacterial plaque and, consequently, the emergence of these pathologies [3].

Tooth decay and gum disease are the pathologies that mostly impact the oral cavity. Thyslstrup and Fejerskov (1995) describe tooth decay as a dynamic process occurring in the bacterial deposits on the dental surface, resulting in an alteration of the oral physiology balance that, along with time, leads to mineral loss. However, it is known that these diseases can be prevented by the adequate mechanical brushing of the teeth associated with a balanced and healthy diet [4].

There are many ways of carrying out actions of preventive approach within the populations. In their studies, many authors [5-7] observe great inefficacy in lectures and specific orientation and suggest that the information must be associated to other interventions, such as applying theories in practice. In view of this, it is observed the need of knowing ways of performing educational activities driven towards this population.

According to Pauleto et al., (2004) [8], the epidemiological situation in oral health is insufficient due to the social and economic conditions of the population, low investment of the public sector, and mainly, the lack of information on basic health care. This condition repeats significantly when it comes to population groups presenting disabilities.

The ones responsible for the person with special needs must be aware of the influence of oral health in the general state of health of these individuals (adapting food and texture for the chewing ability, prevention of aspiration, prevention against infections and endocarditis) and also in the specific place where the problem occurs (local pain, lack of aesthetics, tooth loss) [9]. After all, according to what Oliveira et al., (2007) [10] pointed out, oral problems may involve not only physical health, but also the economic, social and psychological well-being of these individuals. In addition, they can even affect the self-esteem of each one of them, showing the importance of oral health maintenance in the quality of life. For Keye et al., (2005) [11], the caregiver usually does not receive appropriate and sufficient instructions regarding tooth and oral care for the person with special needs, which only increases the risk of this portion of the population to develop oral diseases.

Consequently, oral health education can be a potential instrument in the process of promoting health, because it presents low costs and the possibility of dental impact in the public and collective scope.

Bearing in mind what has been said above, the objective of this study is to assess the effectiveness of different orientation and motivation methods concerning oral health, aimed at individuals with special needs.

MATERIAL AND METHODS

This research was approved by the Research Ethics Committee, number 971.578, and all the participants and/or their caregivers signed the Informed Consent Form and the Informed Acceptance Form. The sample of this study included 21 adult individuals of both genders, average age of 30, with various kinds of disabilities (cerebral palsy, Down Syndrome, intellectual disability and autism), who were employees at the Handicraft Products sector, at the Methodist University of São Paulo.

All individuals went through the clinical oral examination performed by previously calibrated professionals, under natural light, using wooden spatulas, at the beginning of the study and after each motivational intervention. In each examination, the OHI-S Index (Simplified Oral Hygiene Index) was carried out, proposed by Greene and Vermillion (1964) [12] where each tooth surface examined receives a score equivalent to the quantity of bacterial plaque present, and the OHI-S is calculated by the sum of the scores of each evaluated tooth, divided by the number of evaluated surfaces.

Monthly, during 1 academic semester, 4 motivational interventions were carried out with the objective of improving the tooth brushing technique and raising awareness about the importance of the biofilm mechanical removal. After every motivational intervention, a questionnaire to check understanding and comprehension was applied, to evaluate the effectiveness of the performed activity.

The first motivational intervention, *Role-Playing*, was carried out with the objective of clearly explain how and why the accumulation of bacterial plaque happens, and in a playful way, how they could improve tooth brushing, emphasizing the use of dental floss and brushing the tongue as well.

After this activity, a second OHI-S examination was performed. Simultaneously to the examination, the individuals were asked orally at what moment they should use the dental floss, before or after brushing their teeth. Thus, we would be able to evaluate the plot context comprehension. According to the information provided in the role-plays, the individuals should have answered "before tooth brushing."

The second motivational intervention was *Group Dynamics,* where subgroups were randomly divided into 4 groups of 4 individuals, and 1 group of 5 individuals. In this activity, 3 pictures were shown: a person using the dental floss, another one brushing their teeth and a third person brushing their tongue. The objective was that each group agreed among themselves, organizing the pictures in the correct and favorable oral hygiene sequence, putting in first place the dental floss, then tooth brushing and then tongue brushing.

The *supervised brushing* was the third motivational intervention. In this activity, it was observed how individuals used the dental floss, how they brushed their teeth and how they brushed their tongues (Figure 2). The activity was classified as "Good," "Average" and "Bad." "Good," when the individual had sufficient motor skills to carry out the activity; "Average," if the individual showed ability, but with some level of difficulty; and "Bad," if the individual could not carry out the activity.[13] A report was prepared for each individual, containing further orientation.

The fourth motivational activity was a *Lecture for Parents/Caregivers,* where the importance of the autonomy of individuals with special needs was addressed and how to stimulate tooth brushing, as well as information on tooth cavities and gum diseases. In addition, a folder was handed out containing orientation on oral hygiene maintenance along with a report on the difficulties found by each individual and the need of parents/caregivers assisting them to increase their scores.

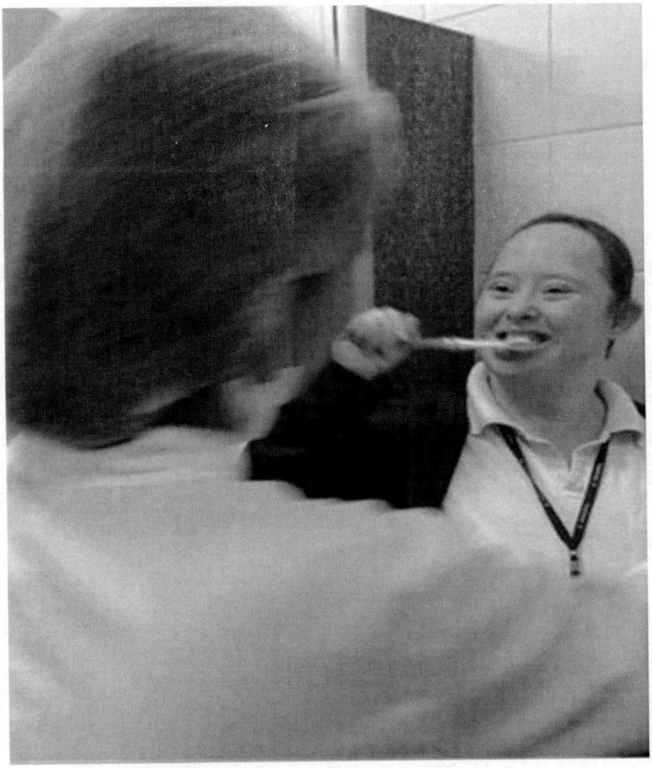

Figure 2. Supervised tooth brushing.

All data was submitted to descriptive and inferential analysis by using the Friedman Test, at 0.05%.

Results

Table 1 describes the number of individuals presenting each kind of disability as well as gender, with Down syndrome being the most frequent pathology, with 9 individuals (42.8%), followed by the Fragile X Syndrome, with 4 individuals (19%).

In relation to gender, 52.4% were women and the average age was 30.

Table 1. Descriptive characteristics of individuals with special needs evaluated according to medical diagnosis (n = sample)

Disabilities	Gender		
	Female	Male	Total
	n	n	n (%)
Autism	-	1	1(4,8)
Schizophrenia	-	1	1(4,8)
Mild intellectual disability	1	-	1(4,8)
Moderate intellectual disability	1	1	2(9,5)
Multiple Alterations	1	0	1(4,8)
Cerebral Palsy	-	1	1(4,8)
Diagnosis not specified	1	0	1(4,8)
Down Syndrome	6	3	9(42,8)
Fragile X Syndrome	1	3	4(19)
Total	11	10	21(100)

The OHI-S indexes during the 5 evaluation moments are shown in Figure 3. Among the first, second and third examinations there was a fluctuation between the "Good" OHI-S score, reaching 90.4% after the 5th motivation. The initial "Average" OHI-S score was of 19.05%, dropping to 4.8% in the end, and there was even an increase in the "Excellent" OHI-S score, from 0 to 4.8%.

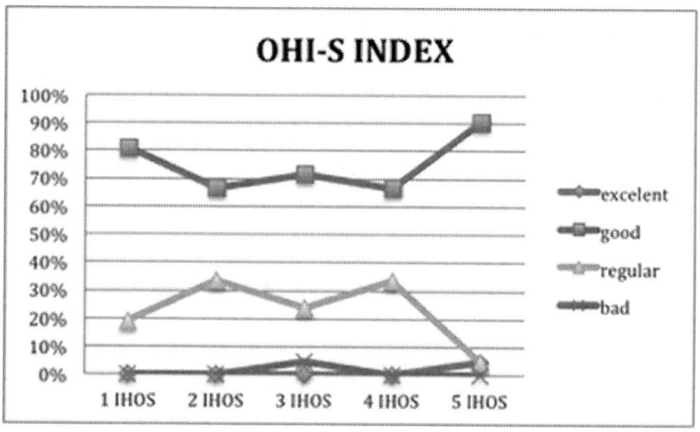

Figure 3. OHI-S index results of the 5 evaluations.

After the first motivational intervention, most individuals understood and assimilated the sequence regarding the use of dental floss; 66.70% reported that they should floss before brushing, 28.60% after brushing, and only 4.80% reported that they use the dental floss before and after brushing.

The evaluation of their comprehension about the correct tooth brushing sequence after the Group Dynamics was understood by only 28.57% of the sample, who stated that they use the dental floss, brush their teeth and then their tongues. In this same activity, it was observed that many individuals would forget to take the dental floss with them. It was also observed that the motor skills were the biggest impairment found, as well as the amount of toothpaste used on the toothbrush.

After the 5th intervention, a Lecture with Parents/Caregivers, 70% of the studied individuals answered the correct sequence of the tooth brushing technique and regarding the number of daily brushings, 85% reported brushing at least 3 times a day: in the morning, in the afternoon and in the evening.

DISCUSSION

Social and family inclusion favors a lot the quality life of the disabled population and, as part of this process, oral health represents an essential aspect in the acceptance of the individual with disabilities by society and in their quality life, since it is associated with a efficiency in his mastication and consequently in his food digestion, improvement in his speech, aiding in communication and a smile-friendly aesthetic that influences self-esteem and contributes to social insertion.

Hogan and White (1982) [14], Stiefel et al., (1984) [5] and Allen et al., (1987) [4] verified a huge decrease in oral problems on patients with disabilities who underwent continuous health education programs. Is also important the effectiveness evaluation of these programs, thus, the biofilm amount evaluation can be a marker of success or not of the educational activity.

The information and education of this population and of those who are responsible for them should always be the first choice so they themselves can raise and improve the level of oral health, which is also the easiest and most economically viable option for health promotion [10].

Individuals with disabilities should be educated in oral hygiene according to their motor skills. The limit of his autonomy for tooth brushing is his efficiency to eliminate dental plaque.

The trained parents/responsible have few problems on tooth brushing their young children, however, adolescents and young adults often want to brush their own teeth and thus may compromise their oral hygiene [3]. In this study the group studied was of adults with a mean age of 30 years, justifying the importance of parent/responsible orientation.

An important factor also observed in this research was the increase in assertions about the contents, when they were individually approached in supervised brushing. In addition, the lecture to the parents/responsible brought an evolution also in the answers of the participants, demonstrating the importance of working with the family when it comes to information that necessarily involves changing habits.

The family participation implied in the tooth brushing quality improvement of the individuals in the sample. Parents and responsible through this interaction promote improvements in the development of autonomy, respecting the limits of each individual. This cooperation, in the process of building this autonomy, causes the individual to change habits, in daily life at home, at work and school, and this is of utmost importance for the improvement of their quality life.

Pauleto et al., (2004)[8] emphasize the need to "replace oral health education models anchored in unidirectional, dogmatic and authoritarian communication practices focused on the transmission of information, through discussion and reflection, triggered by the problematization of oral health themes."

For individuals with special needs, it is essential to use attention-grabbing techniques because they are often scattered and agitated, losing focus quickly. It was observed that after the theater activity most of the individuals answered the evaluation question for the activity understanding, correctly (66.70%) when they stated that it is necessary to floss before brushing. This result was more positive than the question asked after the dynamics groups, in which there was 28.57% of assertiveness.

It is important to emphasize that the use of audiovisual resources, in health education actions may be a factor that arouses the interest of the population, however, attention is required to the periodicity of these interventions so they can be truly effective. Garcia et al., (1998) Marega, Aiello (2015)[15, 16] point out that if these audiovisual resources are associated with interaction with the target population, the results are more positive.

The continuity of the educational process was an important transformative instrument that demonstrated a significant improvement, in the answers obtained on the contents covered during the research, demonstrating a sediment learning that can influence the change in hygiene habits. These data get clear when we observe that, between the last two activities, there was an increase in good and excellent OHI-S scores with a corresponding drop in the regular score.

CONCLUSION

The educational activities regarding oral health for individuals with special needs are efficient in reducing the biofilm when carried out continuously, along with individualized activities.

In patients with special needs, the involvement of the family nucleus is extremely important for the changes in hygiene habits, contributing to the development of the autonomy in the oral health self-care.

Further studies are necessary in this area, once the social group presenting special needs is a diverse group with many variables, and, in addition, shows greater need for projects and public policies to be developed for the improvement of oral health, and, consequently, the promotion of health.

REFERENCES

[1] BRASIL CdC. *Pessoas com Deficiência*. Luzia Maria Borges Oliveira Secretaria de Direitos Humanos da Presidência da República (SDH/PR)/Secretaria Nacional de Promoção dos Direitos da Pessoa com Deficiência (SNPD)/Coordenação Geral do Sistema de Informações sobre a pessoa com Deficiência. [Disabled people. Luzia Maria Borges Oliveira Secretary of Human Rights of the Presidency of the Republic (SDH / PR) / National Secretariat for the Promotion of the Rights of Persons with Disabilities (SNPD) / General Coordination of the Information System on Persons with Disabilities.]2010.

[2] Unidas CRdIdN. Alguns Factores e Números sobre as Pessoas com Deficiência Brussels [Some Factors and Numbers on Persons with Disabilities Brussels]: *URNIC*; 2015. Available from: http://www.unric.org/pt/pessoas-com-deficiencia/5459.

[3] Morgan, J. P., Minihan, P. M., Stark, P. C., Finkelman, M. D., Yantsides, K. E., Park, A., et al. The oral health status of 4,732 adults with intellectual and developmental disabilities. *The Journal of the American Dental Association*. 2012; 143(8):838-46.

[4] Thyslstrup, A., Fejerskov, O. *Cariologia Clinica*. São Paulo: Santos. 1995.

[5] Stiefel, D. J., Rolla, R. R., Truelove, E. L. Effectiveness of various preventive methodologies for use with disabled persons. *Clin. Prev. Dent*. 1984; 6(5):17-22.

[6] Allen, E., Barnes, G., Cole, J., Parker, W., Lyon, J., Armentrout, W., editors. Mental-patients requirements for dental-care-need for preventive programs. *Journal of dental research*; 1987: Amer. Assoc. Dental Research 1619 Duke st., Alexandria, VA 22314.

[7] Milori, S. A., Nordi, P. P., Vertuan, V., Carvalho, J. Respostas de um programa preventivo de placa dentária bacteriana.[Answers from a Preventive Bacterial Dental Plate Program] *Rev. odontol. UNESP*. 1994; 23(2):325-31.

[8] Pauleto, A. R. C., Pereira, M. L. T., Cyrino, E. G. Saúde bucal: uma revisão crítica sobre programações educativas para escolares. *Ciênc saúde coletiva.* [a critical review of educational settings for schoolchildren. Ciênc collective health] 2004; 9(1):121-30.

[9] Faulks, D., Hennequin, M. Evaluation of a longterm oral health program by carers of children and adults with intellectual disabilities. *Spec Care Dentist*. 2000; 20:199-208.

[10] Oliveira, A. C. B., Paiva, S. M., Pordeus, I. A. Parental acceptance of restraint methods used for children with intellectual disability during dental care. *Spec. Care Dentist.* 2007; 27: 222-6.

[11] Kaye, P. L., Fiske, J., Bower, E. J., Newton, J. T., Fenlon, M. Views and experiences of parents and siblings of adults with Down Syndrome regarding oral heathcare: a qualitative and quantitative study. *Br. Dent. J.* 2005; 198:571-8.

[12] Greene, J. C., Vermillion, J. R. The simplified oral hygiene index. *J. Am. Dent. Assoc*. 1964 Jan; 68:7-13.

[13] de Abreu, M. H., Paixão, H. H., Resende, V. L., Pordeus, A. Mechanical and chemical home plaque control: a study of Brazilian children and adolescents with disabilities. *Spec. Care Dentist.* 2002 Mar-Apr; 22(2):59-64.

[14] Hogan, J. I., White, T. Dental health education in an adult handicapped centre. *Dent. Update*. 1982 Jun; 9(5):283-4, 286-8, 290.

[15] Garcia PPNS, Corona SAM & Valsecki Júnior. A educação e motivação: segunda avaliação da efetividade de métodos educativos-preventivos relativos à cárie dental e à doença periodontal. [Education and motivation: second evaluation of the effectiveness of educational-preventive methods related to dental caries and periodontal disease.] *Revista de Odontologia da Unesp.* 1988; 27(2):405-415.

[16] Marega, T., Aiello, A. L. R. Autismo e tratamento odontológico: algumas considerações [Autism and dental treatment: some considerations]. *JBP Rev. Ibero-Am. Odontopediatr. Odontol. Bebê.* 2005; 8(42): 150-7.

INDEX

A

B

C

D

E

F

G

H

I

J

K

L

M

N

O

P

Q

R

S

T

U

V

W

Y